PERFECT *FIT*
COUPLES EDITION

WORKOUTS AND **REFLECTIONS** FOR
A ROCK-SOLID **RELATIONSHIP**

DIANA ANDERSON-TYLER
WITH BEN TYLER

Red Slippers Press

DISCLAIMER

CrossFit® is a registered trademark of CrossFit, Inc. This book was written and published independently of CrossFit, Inc. and is not affiliated with CrossFit, Inc. in any way.

This book contains the opinions and ideas of its author. It is solely for informational, motivational, and educational purposes and should not be used as a substitute for professional medical treatment.

The exercise program within Perfect Fit, or any other exercise program, may result in injury. Consult your doctor before beginning this or any other exercise program. If you begin to feel faint or dizzy while doing any of the exercises in this book, consult your doctor. Like any physical activity involving speed, agility, equipment, or balance, the exercise program in this book poses some inherent risk. The author advises readers to take full responsibility for their safety and know their limits. The author is not responsible or liable for any loss or damage allegedly arising from any information or suggestion in this book.

DEDICATION:

This book is dedicated to our parents, David and Ginnie Tyler and Mitchell and Barbara Anderson. A whole book could be written on how you each have blessed Ben and me with your countless examples of love, humility, compassion, and selflessness. Your prayers for and support of our marriage are inexpressibly precious to us, and we thank God for the values and principles He's instilled in us through you and your beautiful relationship with Him, and with one another.

CONTENTS

INTRODUCTION 1

PROLOGUE: HOW TO USE THIS BOOK 7

PART I: REFLECTIONS 11

Day 1 13
Day 2 15
Day 3 17
Day 4 19
Day 5 21
Day 6 24
Day 7 26
Day 8 29
Day 9 33
Day 10. 36
Day 11. 40
Day 12. 42
Day 13. 45
Day 14. 48
Day 15. 51
Day 16. 54
Day 17. 57
Day 18. 61
Day 19. 64
Day 20. 67
Day 21. 70
Day 22. 74
Day 23. 77
Day 24. 80
Day 25. 84
Day 26. 87
Day 27. 93
Day 28. 96
Day 29. 99
Day 30. 102
Day 31. 104

PART II: PARTNER WORKOUTS 107

APPENDIX A: EXERCISE INSTRUCTIONS 131

APPENDIX B: THE STRETCHES 189

ACKNOWLEDGEMENTS 193

AUTHOR'S NOTE 194

ABOUT THE AUTHORS 195

INTRODUCTION

I feel like I can conquer the world with one hand,
when you are holding the other.

—*Unknown*

Welcome to my very first fitness book that isn't for women only! It's been on my heart for some time to invite our significant others to join us on our adventure of faith-fueled fitness for several reasons.

First, it's not easy to commit to a healthy lifestyle of whole, God-made foods and regular gym time when your spouse insists that potato chips are vegetables and that channel surfing counts as exercise.

Second, staying on track is made much more difficult when you are constantly subjected to your spouse's spaghetti-wrapped fork or ice cream-laden spoon, tempting you to throw your spaghetti squash against the wall and dive into that pint of Rocky Road.

Third, working out becomes infinitely more enjoyable when you are feeling the burn, the sweat, the endorphin rush alongside your "swolemate" (one of my favorite 21st century vocab words).

And last, but not least, there's no motivation quite as powerful and effective as the kind that comes from the one you're married to. Apart from God, our spouse loves us more than anything or anyone else in the world, and when they begin to pursue a fit life with us, they'll be more inclined to pray for and support our physical health as much as they do our mental, emotional, and spiritual wellbeing.

I like to joke that on the first day I met my husband Ben, we were already discussing rings. Granted, they were Olympic rings, but rings—a universal symbol of lifelong love and commitment!—nonetheless. I had been briefly introduced to him earlier that day at a local CrossFit event that my gym was hosting. He was the coach in charge, and I was a CrossFit-avoiding personal trainer just there to cheer on a friend during her first CrossFit experience.

After the event, I returned to the gym (which at that time had a CrossFit section—what I considered a torture chamber—attached to it) to work out, only to be persuaded by a few of the CrossFit fanatics lingering about that I should do a workout with them.

I don't remember the details of the workout, other than the fact that I felt lucky to be alive afterward. I do know that Ben was buzzing around the whole time in a dizzying blur of activity, sort of like the Tasmanian Devil…minus the guttural sounds and excessive slobbering.

Anyway, after I finally completed the workout, and stopped wheezing, I somehow found myself playing around on the Olympic rings, trying to see if I could support myself on them. Ben came over and gave me a few pointers, and even commented that he was impressed to see that I could lower myself down and push myself back up, a.k.a., "dip." Just four months after this initial ring experience, we were engaged, and not only that, but I gave CrossFit a second chance and have no regrets about that decision!

Before CrossFit, I definitely would have deemed myself "fit." I was at a healthy weight again after being anorexic during high school and college, I ate well, was reasonably strong, and had muscle definition. My very first CrossFit experience, the one that gave me nightmares about ferocious, life-choking burpees, proved to me that I wasn't nearly as in shape as I'd thought. So, as I mentioned earlier, rather than swallowing my pride and sticking with CrossFit as a means to become fitter, I grimaced any time I heard the word "CrossFit" and refused to partake of it ever again. But when I fell in love with Ben, my attitude shifted.

Ben listened intently to my complaints about CrossFit: I wasn't good enough, athletic enough, tough enough, etc. He understood perfectly, as he had heard such concerns countless times from many of the people he trained. He helped me realize that just because I had work to do and wasn't a natural-born CrossFit athlete, I shouldn't simply throw in the towel. If I stopped, it would only be due to a lousy attitude, not an incapable body.

Sure, CrossFit would be a challenge, just like any new endeavor, but it would be worth it! I would become stronger, faster, more flexible, more powerful, all-around more fit, as long as I kept at it.

"No discipline is enjoyable while it is happening—it's painful! But afterward there will be a peaceful harvest of right living for those who are trained in this way." —*Hebrews 12:11, NLT*

Because Ben loved me, he encouraged me. He motivated me. He taught me how to modify intense workouts to suit my level of fitness. He held me accountable to my goals. He celebrated with me when I first lifted 225 pounds off the floor. He was happy for me the day I first ran a mile in under eight minutes and when the mention of burpees didn't turn me into Mr. Hyde (I'm actually rather fond of burpees now, believe it or not!). He picked me up when I was having a pity party and helped steer my gaze away from my troubles and back to my Savior.

Adam and Eve were joined together because God's glorious creation was not yet fully "good" without Eve in it. Before I go on, let me make it clear that women were not formed to be men's personal chefs, housekeepers, and secretaries. (Let me say that there is absolutely nothing wrong with any of those roles if they're what God has called you to!) Paul wrote in First Corinthians 11:7 that women are the glory of man! The gift of Eve's creation was delayed only so Adam would be sure to notice it, and be astonished by it. The fact that God assigned Adam to watch an endless parade of animals pass by, two by two, and name them all was sure to make him sit back and wish for his own mate. When Adam woke up to see Eve standing in purest radiance and shameless beauty before him, he found her breathtaking (maybe his breath felt additionally taken because he was missing a rib?) and knew she was the crown of creation.

Check out this awesome passage in Ecclesiastes, penned by the wise King Solomon:

"Two are better than one, because they have a good reward for their toil. For if they fall, one will lift up his fellow. But woe to him who is alone when he falls and has not another to lift him up!" —Ecclesiastes 4:9-10, NIV

Husband and wife are meant to magnify and honor the Lord as human beings wholly surrendered to Him, and to one another. We are our beloved's, and our beloved is ours, says Song of Solomon, and that speaks of our relationship with our spouse, and our relationship with Christ.[1] In marriage, we're to unconditionally and sacrificially love one another, help and serve one another, and lift each other

---

1 Song of Solomon 6:3

up. And more than anything, we're to reflect Christ's eternal, incomparable, unstoppable romance with His bride, the Church.[2]

This precious thing called marriage, this ages-old institution our culture loves to twist and bash and our adversary loves to attack, is a mind-blowing, soul-stirring, world-shaking idea, one conceived by the Creator of the universe Himself. When couples are strong, when they're doing life together with rock-solid faith and fierce devotion, children and communities and whole nations are blessed as a result. But when couples are weak, when they cave to Satan's assaults, give up on God, abandon each other and wave the white flag, families suffer, societies crumble.[3] There's no question why Satan delights in shattering marriages. In so doing, he shatters living portraits of Christ and His beloved.[4]

You may be wondering, "What does fitness have to do with strong marriages?" While the Bible doesn't contain explicit commandments such as, "Thou shalt squat with thy wife," or "Thou shalt not consume Big Macs with thy spouse three nights in a row," it certainly does exhort us to honor God with our bodies, which are dwelling places of the Holy Spirit. If we believe Jesus' words that husband and wife are one flesh, then doesn't it make sense that this "one flesh" should spur itself on toward health and fitness?

Exercise boasts a plethora of health benefits, most of which you're probably well aware, so I won't list them all here. A few examples, though, are decreased stress, better sleep, controlled weight, decreased risk of certain diseases, improved mood, increased energy, and a more active sex life. Read through that list and ask yourself if each one of those things would be welcomed in your marriage. I have a hunch you'll answer "Yes" to all.

---

2 Ephesians 5:28-33
3 *http://thealexanderhouse.org/the-impact-of-divorce-on-our-society/*
   (accessed September 24, 2015)
4 Ephesians 5:32

Simply put, we live in a crazy world, filled with stressors and demonic forces that are vying to drive couples apart. But thankfully, we don't have to be sitting ducks, shaking in our little duck boots as we wait for calamity to strike. We have a whole arsenal of weapons at our disposal, from spiritual disciplines like prayer and praise to physical ones, like proper nutrition and a consistent workout schedule. All we have to do is take up these weapons and wield them, which, as we all know, is easier said than done.

And that's why I'm writing this book. I want to give you and your spouse a resource that will help you grow closer physically and spiritually with devotionals and workouts you can do together in thirty minutes or less.

Ben and I have seen firsthand the power of praying and studying God's Word together in our own lives. We also know how well healthy bodies contribute to a healthy marriage. It is our prayer that with this book, you and your beloved will embark upon a joy-filled journey of enhanced health and unshakable faith, and that you will always trust and believe that when God brought you together, He created a perfect fit.

"As God by creation made two of one, so again by marriage He made one of two." – Thomas Adam

PROLOGUE
HOW TO USE
THIS BOOK

As the title of this book indicates, within these pages you'll find Reflections to strengthen your spiritual muscles, and partner Workouts to pump up your physical ones! As we get started, allow me to explain the structure of the book…

PART I of this book comprises 31 devotionals for you and your spouse to read together. I chose 31, as you might have guessed, because I think it makes perfect sense to dedicate a month of your choice to reading one Reflection a night. (I know, I know, I'm a genius.)

PART II features 24 workouts designed for you and your spouse to do together. (Hurray for endorphins!) The first 12 can be done without any equipment whatsoever, while the last 12 will require a few dumbbells, medicine balls, and such, which I outline below. I chose to include 24 workouts to allow for necessary rest days following the "three on, one off" workout schedule that Ben and I strongly advocate for high-intensity training. Adhering to this method, you and your spouse will work out for three days in a row, then take a day off, and follow this pattern for the duration of the month. Each workout will take between 10 and 30 minutes.

Does this sound like fun? It will be! I highly recommend that you and your spouse talk about and agree on a set time to do these workouts and read the reflections. And then, keep each other accountable! Ask the Lord to help you prioritize this time together as you realize the importance of growing rock solid in mind, body, and spirit as one flesh, united in Christ!

Here's just a bit of info on the equipment we recommend that you purchase—or pull out of the closet or garage!—to help optimize your workouts.[5] You can find all of the following equipment online. If you decide to buy, Ben and I firmly believe that your investment will prove so life-enhancing that you will make lifelong use of this equipment.

ABMAT

The standard sit-up for which you lie flat on your back limits your range of motion, compresses the spine onto the ground, and places you at a relaxed state between repetitions. The AbMat is a nifty little pad that goes beneath your lower back, right above your waistband, to allow you to complete a sit-up's full range of motion and feel a full stretch.

I personally am a fan of the AbMat because it's comfortable and snug under my back and, unlike a towel or other object, it doesn't slide, wobble, or lose its form. If you don't want to purchase one, I recommend using a tightly rolled up towel or small, firm pillow instead. Anything to brace your lower back is better than nothing!

DUMBBELLS

Of course, we all know what dumbbells are, but why have them in our homes? Well, dumbbells are quite simply a workout staple. They are the meat to a treadmill's potatoes. They're the Sonny to the bicycle's Cher. And they've withstood the test of time.

---

5 The only mandatory equipment is a pair of dumbbells and a kettlebell. Modifications are included in each workout for those of you who don't have and/or don't wish to acquire a pull-up bar or plyo box.

The word, "dumbbell," originated in the sixteenth century when novice church bell ringers found they'd better gain some brawn to do their job adequately. To develop their arm strength, the ringers connected a rope to a metal weight and swung it against imaginary bells which produced no sound, hence, it was a dumb bell. In the eighteenth century, "dumb-bells" became the first pieces of home gym equipment, and a hundred years later, the short bar we know today replaced the rope, and rounded weights were attached at either end.

Dumbbells ensure a balanced workout because they effectively train every muscle group. They offer an increased range of motion, guarantee a challenge so you don't plateau, are completely portable, and most importantly, they're affordable.[6]

If you're brand new to weight training, I suggest purchasing two pairs of moderate-weight dumbbells—one for you, and one for your spouse. When they become too light, move up in five or 10-pound increments.

KETTLEBELL

The kettlebell was developed in Russia in the 1700s and used by the Soviet army as part of their physical training (Can you get any more hardcore?). This cannonball-like cast iron device is an incredible tool for developing strength and endurance as each exercise we do with it requires the entire body. Here are a few more facts about your new favorite workout partner:

- Full-body conditioning.
- Because kettlebell training involves multiple muscle groups and energy systems at once, you'll spend less time working out and still get greater results!
- Increased resistance to injury.

6   Info from Diana's book, *Fit for Faith: A Christian Woman's Guide to Total Fitness*

- The ability to work aerobically and anaerobically simultaneously.[7]
- Improved mobility and range of motion.
- Enhanced performance in sports and everyday functioning
- Major calorie burning. (In a recent study conducted by the highly respected American Council on Exercise, participants burned approximately 20 calories per minute—that's 1,200 calories per hour.)[8]

Ladies, I suggest starting out with a 15- or 18-pound kettlebell and working up to 35 pounds as you increase your strength in the coming weeks. Gentlemen, I recommend beginning with a 25- or 30-pound kettlebell and working up to 45 or 50 pounds.

MEDICINE BALL

Medicine balls—med balls, for short—were used even in ancient times to improve fitness, muscular strength and power, and overall athletic ability. Medicine balls are usually just under 14 inches wide and weigh between 2 and 25 pounds. They can be thrown and caught, and are used in a range of exercises and interchangeable routines designed to strengthen and condition every part of the body.

It's important when choosing a ball not to select one that's too heavy for you. You want a weight that challenges you, but also allows you to maintain control and proper form throughout the movements. Ladies, I suggest that you start out with a 10-pound medicine ball, and gentlemen, I recommend 15 or 20 pounds. Use your discretion regarding which size ball to use during partner exercises, which you will come across later in the book!

---

7   While "aerobic" means "with oxygen," anaerobic means "without air" or "without oxygen." Anaerobic exercise is short-lasting, high-intensity activity, where your body's demand for oxygen exceeds the oxygen supply available. The American College of Sports Medicine (ACSM) defines aerobic exercise as "any activity that uses large muscle groups, can be maintained continuously, and is rhythmic in nature."
8   http://www.acefitness.org/getfit/studies/Kettlebells012010.pdf

PART I
REFLECTIONS

DAY 1

"Love is patient, love is kind."

—1 Corinthians 13:4, NIV

I wrote in the introduction that it was Ben's love for me that compelled him to encourage me to stick with CrossFit, a fitness regimen I thought perfectly suitable for *The Avengers*, but not for me. Had it not been for his uplifting words, I would probably still be one of the most unfit fit-looking people on the planet.

Encouragement is a fruit of love. It is an invaluable kindness, one that can restore our hope and coax us out of the dark rain cloud we've curled up under. It reminds us of who we are and what we have in Christ.

But (there's always a "but," isn't there?), encouragement also requires patience, because sometimes the one we're trying to encourage is about as receptive as a rock.

We've all sat on either side of the table. We've been the encourager who can't seem to sing enough happy songs, recite enough scripture, or bake enough cookies to cheer our spouse up. And we've also been the discouraged, gloomy, downcast Eeyore who'd rather be drenched by the rain than warmed by the fire.

In the context of fitness, often the Eeyore, if you will, has fallen off the Eat Right/Exercise Regularly Bandwagon and is moping in the dust of discouragement. As husbands and wives, this is our cue to step in and encourage, to "build one another up," as the apostle Paul wrote, not indignantly wag our fingers at them or give a passive-aggressive sigh when they refuse to go to the gym with us yet again.

Today, ask the Lord to fill you with a loving spirit. Let His Holy Spirit work in you to produce the fruits of kindness and patience so necessary in human relationships, most of all marriage relationships. Thank Him for the countless times He has shown patience and encouraged you, perhaps by His Word or by His hands and feet (the body of Christ), to face the day with renewed confidence and discipline.

The more we reflect on His love, the better we can project His love.

DAY 2

"For physical training is of some value, but godliness
has value for all things, holding promise for
both the present life and the life to come.

—*1 Timothy 4:8, NIV*

Being healthy together is amazing. If you each worked out yesterday and both of you ate more greens and less junk food with few complaints, then you know this to be true. You feel more energized, less cranky, you slept better, you're motivated, and you're even strangely excited about training again tomorrow or trying a new kale smoothie recipe…and it's just Day 2! Crazy, right?! (Okay, you're probably a little sore, too, but that side effect will subside over time, promise!)

These warm, fuzzy, fitness-related feelings are an example, I believe, of one way discipline produces a "peaceful harvest," as Hebrews says.[9] When we commit to a workout schedule despite our excuses, and prepare healthy foods despite the inconvenience,

9   Hebrews 12:11, NLT

we're rewarded with an inner peace and a soul-deep satisfaction that accompanies God-honoring discipline.

But physical training isn't the be-all and end-all of a healthy marriage. Far from it. Today's verse makes it clear that it is *godliness* that carries the most value. After all, there are plenty of couples out there with killer physiques and enviable work ethic who exercise for the sole purpose of bringing honor and glory to themselves, not to God. As Christians, everything we do is to be done "heartily as to the Lord."[10]

To be married couples who are thriving, and not merely surviving, we need to be fit all the way around: mentally, emotionally, physically, but most of all, *spiritually*. Our bodies are simply the vessels God has molded to house the immortal part of us, our souls. It is our souls, comprised of our mind, will, and emotions, that will remain with us throughout eternity. Our bodies will return to dust and be replaced with glorified ones that won't ever need to step foot in a gym or go on a diet, hallelujah! While the Lord desires, and has commanded, that we honor Him by how we take care of our bodies, such obedience is shortsighted if we neglect to grow closer to Him, and to our spouse, outside of the gym.

Today, make it a point to pray with your spouse. Read and meditate on a chapter in Psalms or a parable in the Gospels with them. Read this or another Christian devotional together and talk about how you can apply what it says to your life as individuals and as "one flesh" joined to be a picture of Christ and His bride within your marriage covenant.[11]

"If you have a Bible that's falling apart, you'll have a life that's not."

—*Adrian Rogers*

---

10 Colossians 3:23, KJV
11 Mark 10:8

DAY 3

"Be kind and compassionate to one another, forgiving
each other, just as in Christ God forgave you."

—*Ephesians 4:32, NIV*

Have you ever heard someone say they couldn't wait to get to the
gym so they could burn off some steam? That their husband or
mom or sister or co-worker had ruined their day by something they
said or did and now the only remedy to their frustration is a stress-
suppressing sweat session? (Say that five times fast!) Or maybe
you've seen someone nibbling feverishly on one Butterfinger after
another and when they sense your concern, they confess they've
had it "up to here" with so and so and are snacking to escape their
anxious state, if only temporarily.

Whether you turn to workouts or junk food, mind-numbing
TV shows or thumb-crippling iPhone games, turning to activities
to distract us from our feelings of offense is only a short-lived,
superficial solution. Not long after you get out of the gym or throw
away your last candy wrapper, you'll be left sitting in the same boat
you were in originally: the unnavigable boat of unforgiveness.

Unless you're a hermit, you're going to be around people. And people, by their very nature, will make you upset, sometimes purposefully, sometimes not. And since you're married and, as we've discussed, Satan hates the marriage relationship, it's likely that he will do everything in his power to shoot fiery darts of accusation, offense, anger, and bitterness between the two of you. The longer we hold on to unforgiveness, the longer the enemy is allowed to wreak all sorts of havoc in our marriages as we isolate ourselves from our spouse, the one we're to love sacrificially, unconditionally.

C.S. Lewis wrote something that beautifully complements today's verse: "To be a Christian means to forgive the inexcusable, because God has forgiven the inexcusable in you."

No matter who it is who has hurt, angered, or disappointed you, and no matter what they've done, don't waste a second stewing on the wrong that's been perpetrated. Forgive them, even if they don't ask for your forgiveness. Did the Roman soldiers ask for Christ to forgive them after they nailed His hands and feet to the cross? No. Did the enraged mob or religious leaders ask Him for forgiveness after they mocked Him while He suffered for their sins? No. And still, He asked God to forgive them, "for they [did] not know what they [were] doing."[12]

He forgave the unforgivable. He redeemed the unredeemable, all because He loves us more than we can ever imagine. When we rise up and forgive others, we show them this sort of crazy, illogical, complete and astounding love. We show them Jesus.

"God proved His love on the Cross. When Christ hung, and bled, and died, it was God saying to the world, 'I love you.'"

—Billy Graham

12 Luke 23:34, NIV

DAY 4

"Whoso loveth instruction loveth knowledge:
but he that hateth reproof is brutish."

—Proverbs 12:1, KJV

I had to go with the King James translation of today's verse because it's not every day you come across a word as epic and Shakespearean-sounding as "brutish"! Other versions of the Bible render the original Hebrew word as "stupid," but I personally feel "brutish" makes more of an impact, don't you? "Brutish" is "stupid" taken to the extreme of hard-headedness and irrationality, an extreme I'm sure none of us wishes to reach! (I'm sort of a word nerd if you couldn't tell. My apologies.)

Anyway, I wanted to follow up Day 3's focus on forgiveness with one about correction, because as spouses in a Christ-centered marriage, we're going to be both forgiven and corrected numerous times because our spouse loves us and desires God's best for us. But how many of you can attest to the fact that receiving correction isn't always an easy task, especially when it's coming from the person who knows us better than anyone else on the planet? (I'm raising my own hand right now…)

Why is correction, a.k.a "reproof," so difficult to receive? Because of a fierce little word called "pride."

Pride makes us puff up our chests when our spouse dares call us out on an unhealthy habit. Pride impels us to pout during supper when our spouse begins to offer unwanted advice. Pride inspires us to give our spouse the silent treatment for two days when all they did was correct our push-up form.

Granted, pride rises up even we receive correction from people other than our spouses, but we usually handle it better when it does; we keep the symptoms concealed so as not to appear *brutish* in front of friends, colleagues, pastors, bosses, etc. But pride, whether masked or manifest, is a sin issue we need to deal with in order to mature as children of God, as well as grow into the plans He has for us as husbands, wives, fathers, mothers, teachers, business owners, doctors, you name it.

The next time your spouse (or anyone, for that matter) corrects you—perhaps for overworking yourself, abusing your body in some form or fashion, or neglecting to spend time in prayer or God's Word—consider whether what they are saying is true and necessary, and then (here's the hard part…) graciously *receive* it. Don't become defensive. Don't deflect by turning the tables and correcting your spouse about something, too. Simply acknowledge that what they've said is on target, thank them for loving you enough to confront you about it, and lastly, repent and ask God for the wisdom needed to make lasting changes.

In multiple places, the Bible tells us God disciplines those He loves, and sometimes, He chooses to use those closest to us to do just that.[13]

"Pride is a barrier to all spiritual progress."

—*Harry Ironside*

13 Proverbs 3:12; Hebrews 12:6; Revelation 3:19

DAY 5

"The soothing tongue is a tree of life, but a
perverse tongue crushes the spirit."

—*Proverbs 15:4, NIV*

Yesterday, in Day 4, I wrote about how we can be a humble *correctee*, if you will, that is, the spouse on the receiving end of a reproof. Today, it only seems natural to address the role of corrector, the one correcting or advising his or her spouse on a particular area of concern.

First of all, let's agree that there are indeed multiple wrong ways to correct, and that we are all guilty of demonstrating them. Until we recognize that we have been at fault, we will remain ineffective, frustrated correctors and will most certainly experience strained, even hostile communication within our marriages.

Here's one (fictional) example in which the wife, the corrector, mishandles a conversation with her spouse about the issue of his poor diet while in line for snacks at the movie theater:

WIFE: You're going to have a heart attack any day now if you keep eating the way you do.

HUSBAND: I'm getting Milk Duds and a Coke. I don't do this every day. Besides, we're at the movies—not exactly a whole lot of healthy options here.

WIFE: (takes Ziploc bag out her purse) You could bring your own, like me. See, I brought homemade trail mix. And you *do* eat like that every day. Don't think I don't see those greasy fast food bags in your truck.

I bet that was an enjoyable movie, ha! The corrector's tongue was anything but soothing. On the contrary, she was harsh (bringing up impending death isn't exactly pleasant), gloating, and self-satisfied ("look how good *I* am with my healthy snack!"), as well as accusatory (no one likes to feel like they're married to a private investigator). The word "perverse," which Bible commentators explain means "cross" and "ill-natured," perfectly sums up her tongue; it likely did little to lift her husband's spirit or encourage him to be make wiser food choices.[14]

Here's how that same scenario would have gone had the corrector's tongue been soothing instead of scathing:

WIFE: What are you going to get to snack on, sweetheart?

HUSBAND: I was thinking of getting some Milk Duds and a Coke. What would you like?

WIFE: I brought homemade trail mix in my purse. Would you like to share?

HUSBAND: That sounds good. Probably a lot better for me, huh?

14 http://biblehub.com/commentaries/proverbs/15-4.htm (accessed September 29, 2015)

Beautiful, isn't it? The corrector didn't even have to mention her husband's worrisome health. By asking a simple question, she was able to gently nudge open the door to conversation rather than kick it down. And her loving invitation to share her snack got his wheels turning as he considered his two choices and pondered which was better, both for his wallet and his waistline. Had he declined to share, and proceeded to buy the candy and soft drink, his wife still would have been successful in planting a seed, and hopefully, by watering it with prayer and continued love, patience, and encouragement (see Day 1), he would decide to be healthier very soon.

Throughout your day today, pay special attention to how you speak to your spouse. Are your words gracious and soothing, or grating and spiteful? Are they filled with love and compassion, or with disgust and animosity? If you find that the majority of what you say is "perverse," ask the Lord to cleanse your spirit and purify your heart.[15] Spend time in His Word and let it transform you from the inside out.[16] And then, be amazed as your tongue becomes an instrument of peace instead of a weapon of war.

---

15 Luke 6:45
16 Romans 12:2

DAY 6

"Make a careful exploration of who you are and the work you have been given, and then sink yourself into that. Don't be impressed with yourself. Don't compare yourself with others. Each of you must take responsibility for doing the creative best you can with your own life."

—Galatians 6:4-5, MSG

"Keeping up with the Joneses." It's a real pandemic in today's society. The condition drives us to peer over the fence into our neighbor's yard and yearn for something they have that we don't, whether it's a freshly renovated kitchen, an inviting infinity pool, or a tall, dark, handsome husband. It's the impulse to scroll through Facebook and Instagram, wishing for the job, the physique, the house, the spouse that others have.

The sickness starts subtly, inconspicuously, presenting itself as nothing more than harmless daydreaming. But slowly and surely, it festers and feeds off the attention we give it, growing into something sinister, something deadly, something called *envy*.

Proverbs 14:30 says "a peaceful heart gives life to the body, but envy rots the bones." When we allow our admiration of others' gifts, blessings, beauty, and relationships to morph into jealousy, we stray from our God-carved path in pursuit of someone else's. By complaining and comparing ourselves, and our marriages, to those around us, we show a lack of trust in the One who's promised to prosper us, not to harm us, the One who has entrusted to us gifts as unique as our fingerprints, gifts meant to thrive and flourish for a tailor-made purpose (Jeremiah 29:11, 1 Peter 4:10). Need I remind you that one such gift is your spouse?[17]

Rather than looking at your friend and wishing you had her body, his job, her artistic talent, his sense of humor, etc., praise God for the blessings He's given *you*. Start with His Son, Your Savior, and then move on to your spouse and family. Next, work your way down the list, naming each of your gifts and talents that you know are God-given. Then, focus on doing your best and giving your all in the various roles you play, as a spouse, sister, brother, friend, neighbor, and on and on. The inclination to compare yourself with anyone else will vanish as you feel the satisfaction and security of knowing that God is pleased with you.

"For am I now seeking the approval of man, or of God? Or am I trying to please man? If I were still trying to please man, I would not be a servant of Christ."

—*Galatians 1:10, ESV*

17 Proverbs 18:22

DAY 7

"He trains my hands for battle; he strengthens
my arm to draw a bronze bow."

—*Psalm 18:34, NLT*

"She sets about her work vigorously;
her arms are strong for her tasks."

—*Proverbs 31:17, NIV*

I've selected two scriptures today because, as you can see, one speaks to the fellas and one to the ladies! Each one shows that physical strength isn't just for "American Ninja Warrior" contestants or action stars. It's for every one of us.

Gentlemen, you are to be strong in order to protect and fight for your families and communities. Sure, you're no warrior-king like David was, but you're the head of your home, and as such, the defender of it. Ladies, you are to be strong because heaven knows you have a plethora of responsibilities that require your attention every day. Strong arms for those tasks are an incredible blessing, enabling you to accomplish everything safely, efficiently, and independently! ("Independent Women" by Destiny's Child just popped into my head...)

Being physically fit, I'm sad to say, generally isn't prioritized in Christian circles. Spiritual fitness, yes. Mental and emotional wellness, you bet. But lifting weights, running sprints, or swimming laps seems too worldly, vain, or materialistic to warrant any spiritual merit. After all, Jesus never gave a parable about the importance of deadlifting (although the power of God did lift Him from the dead!), and Paul never wrote a letter to a church chastising them for not obtaining gym memberships. So why write or read a devotional that emphasizes a Christian's need for physical fitness?

You've probably heard of the Mediterranean Diet. It's a way of eating that focuses primarily on plant-based foods, like fruits and vegetables, whole grains, legumes, and nuts. It also limits red meat and prefers fish and poultry as protein sources. It's the way ancient cultures ate, such as the one in which Jesus and the apostles lived. There was no "junk food." There was no such thing as processed food, toxic artificial sweeteners, or drive-thrus.

Along with a naturally healthy way of eating, the people of the Bible were by no means suffering from a sedentary lifestyle. Ladies, read Proverbs 31 and see what this "wife of noble character" was up to. You will see that she was no slouch, and probably had a pretty impressive pair of biceps! And guys, it might surprise you to learn that Jesus wasn't a carpenter in our modern comprehension of the word. The Greek word used in the New Testament is "tekton," which can mean "craftsman," "a worker in wood," or "a ship's carpenter or builder."[18] Men with this occupation would have been the ones to build such grand and spectacular structures as the Temple of the Lord in Jerusalem. Needless to say, they were

18 *https://www.blueletterbible.org/lang/lexicon/lexicon.cfm?Strongs=G5045&t=RSV*
(accessed September 30, 2015)

undoubtedly in excellent shape and worked out hard every day of the week, save for the Sabbath! Another bit of Bible trivia for you: Mary, the mother of Jesus, is said to have walked 12,187 miles by the time she was 50.[19] That's half the distance around the world at the equator!

I give the examples above to illustrate the fact that health and fitness came naturally to those living 2,000 years ago. Only in the last century have we seen the troubling rise in diet-and-exercise related disease and premature death. As Christians, we should lead the way not only in spiritual health, but physical health as well.

> "Dear friend, I hope all is well with you and that you are as healthy in body as you are strong in spirit."
> —3 John 1:2, NLT

What are some steps that you and your spouse can take today to be more like Jesus in the way you eat and exercise? What are some other reasons why it would behoove you to have a strong body as King David and the Proverbs 31 woman did?

19 http://www.blessitt.com/Inspiration_Witness/MilesJesusandMaryWalked/MilesJesusandMaryWalked_Page1.html

DAY 8

"For ever since the world was created, people have seen the earth and sky. Through everything God made, they can clearly see his invisible qualities—his eternal power and divine nature."

—Romans 1:20, NLT

The Book of Psalms is filled with songs that extol God's craftsmanship throughout creation. One of my favorite psalms is Psalm 8:3-4:

*"When I look at the night sky and see the work of your fingers—
the moon and the stars you set in place—
what are mere mortals that you should think about them,
human beings that you should care for them?" (NLT)*

When most of us think of God's majesty displayed in and above the earth, we often envision big, billowing clouds, rising like towers in a ravishing sunset sky, or a cascading waterfall in Hawaii, snowcapped peaks in Colorado, the reflection of a full moon over a motionless lake at midnight. In other words, what we imagine is extraordinary, breathtaking, almost larger than life.

But what if I told you that such epic, Davidic praise, like we read in the Psalms, can be inspired not just by the well-known masterpieces of nature, but by lesser, more mundane, if you will, objects as well, like fruits and vegetables, for example?

You might be thinking to yourself, *Okay, so an apple a day keeps the doctor away, and carrots are good for our vision.* But I don't exactly want to burst into song about them. Well, maybe this little nutrition lesson will change your mind about that…

I took a nutrition course during my last semester of college that taught all about the vital nutrients found in fruits and vegetables, as well as which diseases those nutrients help prevent and which bodily functions they facilitate. While studying for my first exam, I tried to cleverly devise an easy way to memorize which food did what. If only I'd known that many of the answers can be found in the food themselves! It turns out that a food's mere appearance indicates its importance to our bodies. The following chart illustrates a few examples:

FOOD	APPEARANCE	FUNCTION
Tomato	Red, 4 chambers (like the human heart)	Contains lycopene, an inhibitor of heart disease
Walnut	Looks like a brain with a left and right side and upper cerebrum and lower cerebellum. Even the wrinkles on the nut resemble the brain's neo-cortex	Help develop over 3 dozen neuro-transmitters for brain function

Celery, Bok Choy, Rhubarb	Look like bones	These vegetables are 23% sodium, just like bones. A lack of sodium in the diet forces the body to pull it from the bones, weakening them. These foods replenish the body's skeletal needs.
Grapes	Hang in a heart-shaped cluster, and each grape resembles a blood cell	Contain flavonoids and phytonutrients that decrease risk of heart disease
Kidney Beans	A no-brainer, these look like kidneys!	Heal and help maintain kidney function
Sweet Potatoes	Look like the pancreas	Balance the glycemic index within diabetics
Eggplant, Pears, Avocados	Look like a woman's cervix and womb	Balance hormones, help shed unwanted birth weight, prevents cervical cancer. It takes 9 months to grow an avocado from blossom to ripened fruit!
Olives	Look like ovaries	Assist the health and function of the ovaries
Oranges, Grapefruits, other Citrus Fruits	Resemble mammary glands of females	Assist breast health and the movement of lymph in and out of the breasts
Carrots	A sliced carrot looks like the human eye	Greatly enhance blood flow to the eyes

Pretty amazing, isn't it? This knowledge gives us even more motivation to eat salads chock-full of garden goodness and enjoy the sweetness of citrus on sweltering summer days. And how fun to know exactly what your pre-workout orange or post-workout sweet potato is doing for your body, besides providing energy and revving up your metabolism.

Before your next meal with your spouse, thank God for revealing Himself to you not only through the vastness of the stars and the splendor of the galaxies, but also by the very food that you're about to put into your body, the temple of His Holy Spirit.

> "What can be more foolish than to think that all this rare fabric of heaven and earth could come by chance, when all the skill of science is not able to make an oyster."
>
> —*Jeremy Taylor*

DAY 9

"Praise the Lord, my soul, and forget not all his benefits—
who forgives all your sins and heals all your diseases"

—Psalm 103:2-3, NIV

In yesterday's devotional, I wrote about the wonders of God's creation, some millions of miles above our heads, some tantalizing our taste buds on the tip of our tongue. From the Crab Nebula to a snack of cottage cheese and celery sticks, the Lord has made Himself known to us, just as Paul wrote in Romans 1:20. When we stop to consider the work of His hands and the loving way in which He speaks to us through them, we are moved to praise Him. But along with praising Him, we're also to *remember* all He has done—and is doing—for us.

When we lose sight of the ways God has intervened, created, and restored in our lives, the troubles of this world become magnified. The fruits of the Spirit are stifled as weeds of worry take root and proliferate around us, overshadowing our hope and blocking from our vision the very Light that so longs to melt away our sorrows.

Today's verse tells us that not only does God forgive our sins, but He also heals our diseases. I'm sure you would agree that it is easy, as faith-filled Christians, to believe the former part wholeheartedly, but the latter is tougher to accept as our world is filled with suffering, unhealed diseases, and godly people who die too young. And yet, if we believe the biblical accounts of Jesus' miracles and the wonders worked through the early disciples, and if we open our ears, eyes, and hearts to the modern-day miracles that occur every day, we can say with certainty that God, being the same yesterday, today, and forever, unequivocally does heal the sick, give sight to the blind, speech to the mute, and even resurrected life, in a myriad of ways.[20]

As this is a book for married couples, I won't spend time here addressing physical diseases, but relational ones, the ones that Satan relies upon to weaken and ultimately destroy marriages and tear apart families.

Each year, Ben and I attend Family Life's "Weekend to Remember Getaway" to which hundreds of couples come to claim victory for their marriages, in Jesus' name.[21] What blesses us about this weekend the most isn't hearing the speakers, though they are terrific, but listening to the testimonies of husbands and wives whose marriages were on their last legs. In some cases, divorce papers were waiting at home to be signed, and yet they signed up for the conference anyway as a last-ditch effort to witness a miracle. And a miracle is what they got.

Space does not allow me to detail all the miraculous stories of forgiveness, repentance, and redemption we hear about at these

---

20 For more on the topic of miracles, I highly recommend the book *Miracles: What They Are, Why They Happen, and How They Can Change Your Life* by Eric Metaxas
21 For more info, visit *http://www.familylife.com/weekendtoremember2015/about* (accessed October 1, 2015)

life-changing retreats, and honestly, the healings themselves are not the highlights of the weekend. No, the healings are merely signs pointing Ben and me directly to God, straight into His loving embrace where He delights to trade our ashes for beauty, our mourning for joy, and our despair for praise.[22] Listening to others speak of their triumphs against all odds strengthens our souls and realigns our hearts with the will of the Father. We remember all that God has done for us, marvel at His "benefits," as the psalmist wrote, and praise Him for yet unanswered prayers knowing that with Him, the impossible is made possible, and hope is never lost.

"'Humanly speaking, it is impossible.
But with God everything is possible.'"
—Matthew 19:26, NLT

FUN FACT: The Greek word, used in the New Testament, for miracle is *"simaios,"* which means *"sign."*

22 Isaiah 61:3

DAY 18

"Don't be dejected and sad, for the joy of
the LORD is your strength!"

—Nehemiah 8:10, NLT

We all remember the feeling of falling in love. The feeling of weightlessness, giddiness, like all is right with the world. We felt we would gladly drive 10 hours just to spend one with our new flame. We spent hours dreaming up ways to surprise our love with a delivery or roses at their workplace, poems attached to their door, and candlelit dinners prepared by your own two hands, hands which normally avoid ovens and skillets and other kitchen appliances like the plague (or is that just me?). We make our friends nauseated by our constant commentary on last night's date and the recitation of every text message conversation. We joke with our new significant other that we'll probably never argue, and what's up with married couples being so grumpy with each other anyway?

Now, I'm not cynical about love. It has to start in a fairy land of rainbows and butterflies because if it didn't, and we knew from the get-go how challenging relationships would prove to be, we probably wouldn't enter them at all!

There's a proverb that says love and eggs are best when they are fresh. And many people, still relatively new in their marriages, might agree that indeed, their love was best when it first floated into their life, beneficent and wonderful as Glenda the Good Witch. I admit that I, too, maintained that philosophy for many years. But why is that such a prevalent point of view? I believe the answer comes down to two things: immaturity and—are you ready for this one?—...idolatry.

We are born into this world *immature*, a word that by definition means "not ripe, developed, perfected" and "emotionally undeveloped; juvenile; childish."[23] But as we grow up and endure many of life's painful trials and learn many of its lessons, we mature. We grow from our mistakes, accumulate insight on how to succeed (and fail) at various endeavors, and acquire wisdom that we'll carry with us the rest of our lives.

Generally speaking, it is through firsthand experience that we mature—not through osmosis, and not by vicariously living through movies and books. Until we've been in relationships that have traversed both valleys and peaks (not necessarily romantic ones, but friendships and familial relationships as well), most of us will go through life with an unrealistic, Disneyfied notion of what true love looks like. At the outset, we'll be happy as a diner at IHOP whenever his bacon, pancake stack, and fresh eggs arrive, but if we detect a sour taste or bite into something unsavory, we'll retreat and conclude that Mr. or Mrs. Right is still out there. This is immature thinking.

The second reason why I think many people (including me, at one time) have a negative opinion on the ardor and passion of long-lasting relationships, and marriages in particular, is because we make an idol of our mate. Forgive me, but when I think of a person who depends on his or her spouse for happiness and a sense of self-worth, I think of Max the Weiner Dog. Let me explain.

Max belonged to Mrs. Sabota, the mother of my best friend growing up. Max is the only dog I've ever met who didn't much care for people, except for Mrs. Sabota. (I am a dog lover, by the way, but this pup even I could not love!) He was her dachshund-sized shadow when she was at home, following her from room to room, getting underfoot in the kitchen, rushing up the stairs behind her when she brought snacks up to my friend and me, and barking when unfamiliar people got too close to her. And when she'd leave for errands, he went berserk. He'd scratch at the door and whimper until he got tired, then he'd lie down in front of it, not once moving to get food or water. He definitely could not be consoled by another canine playmate or sympathetic human.

Mrs. Sabota was Max's idol. The only time he was with happy and expressed joy was in her presence. Apart from her, he was a nervous wreck, a depressed mess of a "man's best friend." I'm afraid that he makes an apt metaphor for how we can be when we place our spouse on a pedestal and look to them to be our source of contentment.

Looking back up at our verse of the day, from whom, according to the Bible, are we to derive our strength? From whom are we to receive joy?

The answer: the Lord.

Today with your spouse, discuss this topic of immaturity, idolatry, and contentment and how it relates to your marriage. Talk about how each of you has grown since your relationship began, and in what ways. Be honest about how you can seek joy *not* in one another, but in the King of Kings, the Prince of Peace, our Wonderful Counselor, Jesus Christ.

What is one thing you can start doing today that will bring you closer to Him, the One who created you, the One who knows the number of hairs on your head, and loved you enough to give His life for you?[24]

When you put Jesus first and find your joy in Him no matter the circumstances, you will be amazed at how your marriage flourishes and thrives as a result.

"I pray that God, the source of hope, will fill you completely with joy and peace because you trust in him. Then you will overflow with confident hope through the power of the Holy Spirit."

—*Romans 15:13, NLT*

24 Luke 12:7

DAY 11

"Let him kiss me with the kisses of his mouth—for your love is more delightful than wine."

—Song of Solomon 1:2, NIV

If you really want to know what God's view of love and intimacy is, look no further than Old Testament book, Song of Solomon. It is full of beautiful poetry and vivid imagery of the passionate romance shared by King Solomon and his bride, the Shulammite woman who is never named. The book celebrates marital love in no uncertain terms. In fact, its description of erotic love is so clear and intense that I pity the preachers who have to stand in front of congregations to preach about it while trying not to blush.

The book serves a few key purposes, but I'll only focus on one for the purposes of today's reflection, and that is that it teaches us God's divine design for marriage and the significant role sexual intimacy plays in it.

Song of Solomon shows us that sex is not only a procreational activity, but a recreational and ministerial one as well. The apostle Paul reiterates this concept in 1 Corinthians 7 when he writes that husband and wife are to be intimate together, an exception being if they mutually decide to abstain for a while for the sake of devoted prayer.

In both Song of Solomon and the passage in 1 Corinthians 7, we find that sex, the way God intends is, isn't about *getting* for our own pleasure, but *giving* for the pleasure of our spouse.

Acts 20:35 quotes Jesus when it says that it is more blessed to give than to receive, a teaching that flows consistently throughout the whole canon of scripture. While it may seem counterintuitive, this approach to intimacy, and marriage in general, actually heightens one's experience rather than diminishing it. Have you ever been more excited about giving a gift than the recipient was about opening it? Well, sex with a giving attitude is sort of like that; you'll be just as satisfied to bestow pleasure than to receive it, if not more so.

I'm no marriage counselor or expert on the subject, but I *can* counsel you to reach for your Bibles and perhaps a biblically based study for more insight on sexual intimacy. I hope that today you will be encouraged to view sex as an opportunity to lavish love on your spouse, and in so doing, reflect on earth the heavenly and eternal truth of Christ's fervent, fierce, and glorious love for us, His beloved bride.

PS: Sex can make for a good cardio session, too…

"Done well, marital sexuality can be a
supremely healing experience."

—Gary Thomas

DAY 12

"Look carefully then how you walk, not as unwise but as wise,
making the best use of the time, because the days are evil."

—Ephesians 5:15-16, ESV

The Greek word used for "evil" in today's verse translates to
"hurtful, i.e., evil in effect or influence."[25] When Paul wrote to the
early church in Ephesus, the influence of the culture in those days
(approximately 60-61 A.D.) certainly was evil. It was in Ephesus
where one of the Seven Wonders of the ancient world, the Temple
of Artemis, stood, which was a colossal epicenter for idol worship.
Loose conduct and licentiousness were also pervasive in the city,
as was demonism and sorcery, no doubt a result of the rampant
idolatry that polluted the community with the stench of Satan.

The days have been evil since Adam and Eve gave in to the
serpent's temptation and took a bite from that infamous piece of
fruit. The days were once so evil, in fact, that God had no other

choice but to destroy the earth with Noah's flood, sparing only two of each kind of animal and eight righteous individuals. But that cataclysmic event didn't quell humanity's devilish bent. On the contrary, numerous yet-to-be-fulfilled biblical prophecies foretell another time of unprecedented judgment that will mark the end of this world as we know it.[26]

Today, in 2016, evil has made even more inroads into our lives through the advent of the Information Age and constantly advancing technology that brings the world and all its enticements straight to our fingertips. Movies, music, TV shows, computers and smartphones have the capacity to introduce all manner of evil into our lives, from debauchery and drunkenness to profanity and porn. All the enemy needs is one small crack in our spiritual armor to send an onslaught of arrows whizzing our way, each one tipped with fire and aiming to kill. All he needs us to do is stumble once, make one misstep; then he can send his dark armies after us with snares, temptations, and even doubts about what God says in His Word as he did with Eve in Eden and with Jesus in the wilderness.[27]

So how do we combat this influx of evil? Let's take a look at what follows today's verse:

"Therefore do not be foolish, but understand what the will of the Lord is. And do not get drunk with wine, for that is debauchery, but be filled with the Spirit, addressing one another in psalms and hymns and spiritual songs, singing and making melody to the Lord with your heart, giving thanks always and for everything to God the Father in the name of our Lord Jesus Christ

—Ephesians 5:17-20, ESV

First, we're to know the Lord's will, which we find as we seek Him in prayer and stillness and listen for His voice. And we search

---

26 See 2 Peter 3:8-10, 1 Thessalonians 1:9-10, Acts 17:31, 1 Corinthians 15:23-24, 2 Thessalonians 1:6-7.
27 Genesis 3:1; Matthew 4:1-11

His Word for living, active, penetrating truths that guide our every step like lamps to our feet.[28] Second, we're to be filled not with wine, but with the Spirit and thanksgiving. In other words, we're not to find our joy or solace in anything that would take the place of God in our lives. Instead of pouring wine into our cups, why not pour out upon others the cheer and contentment, praise and peace that accompanies our relationship with Christ? When you have these things, what need is there to reenact a country music video by drowning your sorrows and hurt in alcohol?

Christian husbands and wives (that means you!) are always in Satan's crosshairs, not just because we're Christ-followers, but because we're a picture of Christ's relationship with His Church. If Satan can muddy our white wedding garments and strategically conspire to make us renounce our marriage oath, he can lead the disbelieving world to mock and scoff and claim that our faith is powerless. This is why we're to be wise, ever aware of where we walk, how we talk, and what we see and hear. Ever dressed in the armor of God from head to toe. Ever mindful of the weightiness of marriage and the cosmic significance it bears. Ever thankful for the calling of God on our lives to be salt and light and image-bearers of His Son.

> "Whatever their bodies do affects their souls."
>
> —C.S. Lewis, *The Screwtape Letters*

28 Hebrews 4:12; Psalm 119:105

DAY 13

"O Lord, you are so good, so ready to forgive, so full of
unfailing love for all who ask for your help."

—*Psalm 86:5, NLT*

We all know the story of David and Bathsheba. King David, the
man known for slaying Goliath and chasing after God's own heart,
goes wandering out onto his roof one evening and sees a woman
bathing. He is so arrested by her beauty that he immediately finds
out who she is, and despite learning that she is a married woman,
has her brought to him.

When Bathsheba informs David that she is pregnant, he calls in
her husband, a warrior named Uriah, and subtly encourages him
to go sleep with his wife, even getting him drunk. Uriah, however,
a loyal and honorable soldier, will not enjoy such pleasure while his
comrades are camped out on the battlefield. And so, David's clever
plan to cover up his sin is thwarted.

But David is determined, and desperate. His foolishness has
made him more reckless, more careless. He orders the leader of his

army to place Uriah in the front line of a fierce battle, and then to withdraw from him, thus guaranteeing his slaughter.

After Bathsheba's mourning period has ended, David has her brought to him again and marries her. The King has successfully hidden his sin from the world, but not from God, who sees everything.

God sends the prophet Nathan to recite back to David exactly what he had done, proving without question that David's actions were no secret to the Most High. Instead of blame-shifting, excuse-making, or rising up in anger and having Nathan killed on the spot, David owns up to his sin, declaring, "I have sinned against the Lord."[29]

No one could have accused God of wrongdoing had He chosen to slay David. It was what he deserved for taking the life of an innocent man. But when David, in humility and with genuine remorse, confessed his sin, he was met not with a sword of justice, but the garland of grace. Nathan replied to David, "The Lord also has put away your sin; you shall not die."[30]

Now there were consequences for David's sin. For example, the child he'd conceived with Bathsheba died after his birth. And, as Nathan prophesied, David's household was visited by violence and unrest. Bathsheba, despite being wed to the King, lived in disgrace because of the loss of her child, which in those times, was a sign of the Lord's judgment and disfavor.

One of my favorite verses in the Bible says, "where sin increased, grace abounded all the more."[31] Yes, there were serious consequences for David's sin, but God's love for David and His future plans for Israel could not be stopped. David and Bathsheba (who, one would infer was able to reconcile with David despite his sins) had

29 2 Samuel 12:13a
30 2 Samuel 12:13b
31 Romans 5:20, NASB

Solomon, the wisest king to ever rule and who wrote many of the proverbs, Ecclesiastes, and Song of Solomon.

The repaired relationship between David and Bathsheba is quite miraculous, if you ask me. It shows us that with the Lord's intervention, hardened hearts can be softened, bitter attitudes sweetened, and hopeless outlooks brightened with just a touch of His grace.

All of us have stumbled and fallen short. All of us have had metaphorical blood on our hands and lust in our hearts. But what the story of David and Bathsheba illustrates so powerfully for us is that God does not condemn us without first moving mountains to try and save us. He wants so much to show us the depths of His mercy and the wonder of His forgiveness.

If there is some wrong in your past that has been haunting you, some sin that has driven a wedge between you and your spouse and your relationship with God, surrender it to the Lord. He already knows what you've done. He saw it plainly. And despite all He has seen in your life and mine, He isn't perched high on a cloud with a scowl on His face and a lightning bolt in His hand, waiting for the right time to smite you. Rather, He is just a prayer away, eager to hear the sweet sound of a confession on your lips as you express heartfelt repentance for what you've done. Then, and only then, can He begin the process of restoring your life and refreshing your soul.

> "I learn from the Scriptures that repentance is just as necessary to salvation as faith is, and the faith that has not repentance going with it will have to be repented of."
>
> —Charles Spurgeon

DAY 14

"Forget the former things; do not dwell on the past."

—Isaiah 43:18, NIV

Perhaps the greatest example of total, genuine, no-looking-back forgiveness is found in the parable of the Prodigal Son. We all know the story: Son leaves home. Son squanders inheritance. Son regrets decisions and longs for home. Son returns home and is accepted by father with loving arms.

We're rightly taught in Sunday school and sermons that this parable illustrates our heavenly Father's extravagant love for us. No matter how far we've wandered astray, no matter how often we've refused to heed His word, all of it is in the past, forgotten the moment we run back into His embrace and humbly ask for forgiveness.

But in addition to showing us the loving, merciful, gracious character of God, this story serves as an example of the standard we're called to when it comes time to forgive those who have wronged us, abandoned us, or both. We're shown what love in action looks like.

We're all familiar with 1 Corinthians 13, a.k.a., "The Love Chapter." Many of you probably had it read by someone at your wedding. In case you need a refresher, here's the popular passage:

"Love is patient and kind. Love is not jealous or boastful or proud or rude. It does not demand its own way. It is not irritable, and it keeps no record of being wronged. It does not rejoice about injustice but rejoices whenever the truth wins out. Love never gives up, never loses faith, is always hopeful, and endures through every circumstance."

— *1 Corinthians 13:4-7, NLT*

For the purposes of today's reflection, I wish to highlight the words, "it keeps no record of being wronged." I don't know about you, but showing love this way does not come naturally for me! When I am operating by the flesh and not walking by the Spirit, the second Ben does something to irk me, I am prone to rattle off a litany of his past wrongs more precisely than I can recite the ABCs.[32] "You tracked in dirt through the house again, Ben. You did that last Tuesday, and the Thursday before that! I stepped on a sticker bur today, thank you very much! By the way, you owe me an apology for forgetting to give me a Valentine's Day card four years ago."

Okay, so I exaggerated a bit at the end, but you get my point. How quickly we can take a current hurt or vexation and treat it like a starting gun. No sooner do we feel offended than we take off racing around the track of undealt-with anger, bitterness, and a boatload of grudges. Needless to say, this is not the way to handle offense of any kind.

32 Galatians 5:16

Jesus gave the commandment to love one another, just as He has loved us.[33] Like God the Father, of whom Jesus is the express image, we are to exhibit love in all circumstances, even when it comes to forgiving those who have wounded us.[34] Even when it comes to accepting a spouse who has broken our heart.

Today, ask the Holy Spirit to grow in you the fruits of patience and self-control so that you, like the father of the Prodigal, will leave the sins and grievances of the past behind and love others as God loves you.

"I am amazed by how many individuals
mess up every new day with yesterday."

–Gary Chapman

33 John 13:34
34 Hebrews 1:3

DAY 15

"Dear brothers and sisters, when troubles of any kind come your way, consider it an opportunity for great joy. For you know that when your faith is tested, your endurance has a chance to grow."

—James 1:2-3, NLT

As someone who's been both a Christ-follower and a fitness fan for quite some time now, I can't help but create a few faith-related metaphors from the world of weightlifting, running, jumping, rowing, and, to put it plainly, *suffering* for the greater good! (For the record, if anyone tells you working out is easy, they're selling you something. It's called *working* out for a reason!) Here are a few analogies I've formed over the years:

* Warmup is to workout as this earthly life is to eternal life[35]
* Resistance training is to body as trials are to spirit
* Healthy food is to body as God's Word is to soul

---

35 For more on this analogy, check out my blog, *http://www.dianaandersontyler.com/high-knees-and-heaven-the-power-of-the-warm-up/*

The second one is the one I will flesh out in today's reflection, because I think it will serve us well in our marriages as we face spiritual, emotional, and mental "resistance" whether from the world, the enemy, or our own flesh.

We can all easily name sources of marital strife, for example, financial strain, infidelity, constant criticism from one or both spouses, a lack of passion, and the list goes on. These "resistors" can wear and tear at relationships over time until "enough is enough," and someone collapses beneath the weight of them, thus ending the marriage.

I love this famous quote from Winston Churchill: "If you're going through hell, keep going."

Why, we might ask Mr. Churchill, should we keep on going through hell? Hell is hot. Hell is full of torment and agony. Why not turn around and hightail it out of there?

It was Mr. Churchill's courageous attitude and resolve to "never, never, never give up" that led the British people to victory during World War II. It's the same attitude that drove Caleb to declare to Moses regarding the Promised Land, "Let's go at once to take the land! We can certainly conquer it!"[36] Even though his comrades were scared to death to fight the giants who made them feel like "grasshoppers," Caleb had faith in the God who had led them this far and refused to back down.

Churchill's confidence to advance against fear and defy the odds didn't come from nowhere. He had been kept out of politics for two years and taught himself how to paint to escape the doldrums. In 1922 he lost his seat in Parliament while hospitalized with acute appendicitis. But he didn't wallow in self-pity. Instead, he wrote his monumental six-volume work on World War I called *The World Crisis.*

Churchill regained his seat in Parliament, but did not hold a major government position for 10 years. He continued to write, finishing a number of books, kept giving speeches, and carried on with painting and even learned how to lay bricks. In 1940, King George VI asked Churchill to be the next Prime Minister at a time when his country needed him most. His perseverance through life's difficulties had proven to him that disappointments and setbacks don't mean the end of the world. Rather, they're opportunities to grow, to rest, and to wait for the One who loves us most to direct our steps at the proper time, and to lead us to doors we never would have found had hardships not altered our course.

Getting back to workouts… We know they're challenging. They burn, make us sweat, and take time out of our day. But the rewards they produce are more than worth the effort. Exercise prevents heart disease, diabetes, and other diseases. It increases our energy, improves our sleep, along with a host of other things that you can Google if you have any doubts. But these benefits don't occur overnight. (If they did, there wouldn't be enough gyms to facilitate all the people wanting to use them!) But for those who are patient, persevering, and self-disciplined, the results *do* come with time. Unfortunately, too many of us abandon the gym much too early, never experiencing the awesome improvements in strength, mood, libido, and so many other things.

It's the same with marriage. The struggles are our barbells. The rough patches are our uphill sprints. But if we echo Churchill and "never, never, never give up," no matter how heavy and hard the resistance, we will emerge stronger, happier, better equipped, more confident, and, truthfully, more in love than ever.

"Soul mates are not found, they are formed."

—*Brian Donovan, Marriage Counselor*

DAY 16

"So he got up from the table, took off his robe, wrapped
a towel around his waist, and poured water into a basin.
Then he began to wash the disciples' feet, drying them
with the towel he had around him."

—John 13:4-5, NLT

A few weeks ago, Ben and I saw the movie *War Room*, which became an immediate all-time favorite. (If you haven't seen it, I highly recommend you schedule a night in and rent it…or better yet, buy it!) It's about a married couple, Tony and Elizabeth, who, from the outside looking in, seem to have it all together. But the reality is, their marriage is falling apart. Tony has become work-obsessed and preoccupied with a pretty colleague. Elizabeth's bitterness has increased while her hope in restoring their marriage continues to nosedive.

When Elizabeth meets Miss Clara, she's challenged to set up her own "War Room," that is, a closet devoted solely to steadfast, heartfelt prayer and meditation on God's Word. Elizabeth learns that victories aren't handed to us. We must fight for them.

Elizabeth and Tony's battle isn't won overnight, but by the grace of God and with no shortage of patience and prayer, the couple comes together with contrite hearts and surrendered spirits, ready to enter a season of divine healing.

The scene in the film that clearly shows that Tony isn't the same man he was when it began is one in which he totally surprises his wife—and the audience—by fulfilling two of her greatest wishes: a decadent ice cream Sunday ("Hot fudge everywhere and lots of whipped cream") and a foot rub (it should be noted that her character is known to have stinky feet!). Can any of you ladies relate to those desires?

When Elizabeth first made these wishes known to Tony when he asked her, "What do you want?" over dinner one night, he almost winced at the notion of touching her feet. Needless to say, he didn't budge to buy her a sundae, either. But on this occasion toward the "happy ending," Tony seems eager, giddy even, to pamper his wife. Just after he asks her to sit on the sofa and serves her a mouthwatering mountain of an ice cream sundae, he brings out a bucket of water and proceeds to scrub and rub her feet, albeit, while wearing a surgical mask to keep the smell at bay.

Watching this scene, I, and likely millions of other audience members, couldn't help but be reminded of one the most marvelous acts of Jesus in all of the New Testament: the washing of His disciples' feet. This act was a servant's job, and by no means fit for a rabbi like Jesus, much less the Savior and Creator of the world. Moreover, do you know how filthy people's feet were back then? The roads they walked miles and miles on were dusty, and this was long before Nikes and Adidas were invented, and I'm not sure about pedicures... Suffice it to say, feet simply weren't features one would brag about, or want their beloved teacher, Lord, and friend to wash.

But Jesus wasn't above washing sandy, rough, callus-covered feet. In fact, it was His intention to bring Himself low. This great act of humility demonstrated to His followers, and to you and me, how we are to serve others with a lowliness of heart and mind that is incredibly rare, if not non-existent, apart from the regenerating work of the Holy Spirit in our lives. This remarkable principle of putting others' needs before our own and thinking of them more highly than we think of ourselves is found over and over again in Scripture; it's one we would be wise to apply to our marriages every day, as God always rewards obedience with blessing and proves to us how much more blessed it is to give than to receive.

How can you astound your spouse with an unexpected act of humility and love today?

"Do nothing from selfish ambition or conceit, but in humility count others more significant than yourselves."

—*Philippians 2:3, ESV*

DAY 17

"The seed that fell on the footpath represents those who hear the
message, only to have Satan come at once and take it away."

—Mark 4:15, NLT

Have you ever heard a wonderful, hard-hitting sermon, one that
made you laugh, cry, jump up and down, lift your hands, and
shout "amen" because of how penetrating it was or how perfectly it
spoke to your circumstances? Those are powerful hours. We walk
out of the sanctuary and smile at the sunshine as though beholding
it for the first time. The green grass glows and the birds chirp
harmoniously as we take in the sweet air of hope and excitement
and exhale the doubts and dread that have hitherto worn us down.
The future is bright and the past can't hinder us any longer.

Okay, now for a second question: Have you ever been strolling
happily along a week or so after your "Aha moment" in church
when all of a sudden, you come under a spiritual attack? But it's not
just any spiritual attack. It's a very strategic and specific one, aimed
against the very issue you celebrated finally facing and defeating in
the pew or at the altar just days before. At that time, you felt on

top of the world, invincible, as if you'd never wrestle Issue X again. But now, you're lying flat on your back in the metaphorical mud of discouragement while the rains of condemnation pour down on you. "What happened?" you think. "I thought I was past this…"

What happened is Satan's minions—the birds, as the verse in Mark 4 calls them—carried the transformative word away.[37]

Satan has an untold number of beady, black, and evil-filled eyes observing God's children, waiting for an opportunity to wreak havoc and cause chaos. Like a swarm of vicious hawks and hungry vultures, they're circling over our heads in the invisible war zone around us, hunting for moments of weakness, eager to incinerate moments of strength.

What Satan and his armies hate most, apart from souls accepting Jesus as Lord and being rescued from the bondage of sin and death, is when God's children make spiritual headway, because that means they're becoming more Christlike, and therefore, a greater threat to their kingdom of darkness. So, as soon as they see that we've experienced a divine revelation, something that could change our attitude, our job, perhaps our whole life for the better, they will swoop down and snatch away the seed, that is, the word of God, before it takes root in our heart.

This has happened to me on numerous occasions. For example, after listening to an excellent podcast on prioritizing time with your spouse, I was stoked and super-motivated to set aside a few hours each night, no matter what writing work was left undone, just to be with Ben.

You see, as a self-employed writer, I keep odd, often sporadic hours, to say the least, while my husband works a steady schedule. At the time of this example, he was getting off work around 5, while I would write until 7 or 8, leaving just an hour or two for

---

37 In the Bible, birds often represent Satan.

"us time." This bothered him, understandably, but in the name of self-discipline and diligence, I made excuse after excuse for why I couldn't just stop writing—I simply wasn't at a stopping place. But after I heard this podcast, I realized that my priorities needed to shift. Ben needed to be at the top again, right after God.

Satan didn't like this, by any means. Like I've written in previous reflections, he despises Christian marriages, so anything that keeps us apart from our spouse he celebrates. The very night on which I was going to change my tune and shut down my laptop when Ben walked in from work, the old excuses for why I needed to keep working started popping up and taking over. It was as if I'd forgotten all about the message I'd heard and the resolution I'd made to devote time to Ben in the evenings. Things didn't change for some time until again, by God's grace, He dealt with me on this issue and I realized my previous mistake…

You might have noticed that I said "*I made*" the resolution to change. In other words, I was relying on my own self-effort and will to be a more loving and selfless spouse. This gave the devil's predatory birds the opportunity they needed to steal the precious seed right out from under me. The soil of my heart was not able to receive the seed because it was filled with self-centeredness.

Later on, when I humbled myself before the Lord and repented of my hardened heart and its impenetrable soil, the enemy no longer had a stronghold. I knew that by submitting to the Lord, trusting Him to transform me from the inside out, and covering myself with the armor of God, Satan was no match for me. That's not to say he or his soldiers won't make their rounds, but when they do, I'll be ready to fight back and send them retreating back to where they came from.

"Submit yourselves, then, to God. Resist the devil,
and he will flee from you."

—James 4:7, NIV

How is the soil in your heart? If it needs softening or nourishing, don't go to a book (unless it's the Bible!), a conference, a motivational speaker or friend, your spouse, or your own strengths to change it. Go to the Lord. Ask Him to garden it in the ways only He can. Let Him prune, plow, till and plant so that He can pour His life-giving, soul-refreshing seed into your heart. You will be amazed at the harvest He produces!

"I am the true vine, and my Father is the gardener."

—John 15:1, NIV

DAY 18

"Understand this, my dear brothers and sisters: You must all be quick to listen, slow to speak..."

—James 1:19, NLT

In yesterday's devotional, I wrote about an area I struggled with in my marriage, namely an obsession with work that kept me from spending invaluable time with my husband. So, I thought it only fair to pick on him for today's reflection, ha! But in all seriousness, I believe it will be helpful for you all to read this– especially you guys out there—because I have a feeling you'll relate. Just promise me you won't point fingers at one another and say, "You do that, too!" With the Holy Spirit's help, your spouse will be able to pick up on what he or she needs to correct, and you can sit back and relax, knowing God's taking care of it.

Besides owning our CrossFit gym, Ben is a mechanical engineer for an oil and gas company here in San Antonio. Needless to say, he is what they call, "left-brained." In fact, sometimes I wonder if his brain even has a right side! (Kidding, kidding…) Anyway, when it comes to what God has called him to do, both in owning and running a business and designing and building things like vessels, piping, pumps, and electrical systems, Ben has got the intellectual goods. He's analytical, logical, decisive, and loves to problem solve. However, these awesome qualities, which serve him well in work, haven't always been so awesome when it comes to comforting and encouraging his wife...

A few months ago, I was sitting on the couch feeling rather glum when Ben came home from work and could see that I was distraught. He sat down beside me and asked what was wrong. I was looking at a quote on a book cover I'd received from a designer, and the price was more than I'd anticipated and definitely out of the budget Ben and I had set for this project. I explained to Ben that everything else for the book—the editing, layout, formatting, etc.—was in place, and that the cover was to be the icing on the cake. After all, it is one of the most important aspects of a book, as it is what grabs readers' attention. But this icing, unfortunately, was out of our price range.

Ben will admit that fixing broken things is a bit of a reflex for him. He's good at it, and he enjoys it. Just last night he went over to fix a friend's motorcycle and came home grinning that he'd gotten the job done. Over the weekend, he fixed some computer issues my mom was having and even calculated how much money she would save each month if she switched to using LED lightbulbs. The man loves to help, and it's one of the God-given qualities in him that I love most.

What I wanted at that day on the couch, and what I needed, was a listening pair of ears. I didn't want to solve the problem or have someone fix it. I wanted to be encouraged so that I wasn't focusing on it anymore. I had worked so hard on this book, my first novel, and felt like I had hit a wall. I wanted it to look as eye-catching as possible and knew the company I had sought out would do a fantastic job.

Ben reacted, understandably, by wanting to *fix* instead of focus on what I was feeling. No sooner had I showed him the invoice than he began rattling off ideas on how I could design the cover myself. His suggestions weren't all bad, I must say, but at the time, they only overwhelmed me more. Each one was translated in my head as "More work! More time! And I'm *soooo* not qualified!" My eyes began to water with frustration and anger that he wasn't helping, though he thought he was being extremely helpful.

Today's verse tells us to be quick to listen and slow to speak, and I can think of no other context for which this precept is more important than the marriage relationship. As husbands and wives, we are going to experience countless ups and downs in life, conflicts and disappointments that will scare, shake, and stymie us. When those trials beset us, what we need, more than anything, is our spouse's hand to hold, our beloved to talk to, cry on, and confide in.

Be that hand and that pair of ears for your husband or wife the next time they're having a bad day or a dark hour. The time will come for you to present your ideas for solutions, but don't rush it. Ask God to help you be a reflection of who Scripture says He is to us when we are dismayed: a strong tower, a refuge, a shield.[38]

"I'll lift you and you lift me, and we'll both ascend together."

—*John Greenleaf Whittier*

38 Proverbs 18:10, Psalm 46:1, Proverbs 30:5

DAY 19

"I also tell you this: If two of you agree here on earth
concerning anything you ask, my Father in heaven will
do it for you. For where two or three gather together
as my followers, I am there among them."

—*Matthew 18:1-20, NLT*

One of the best compliments I've ever been paid was given by my
husband just two weeks ago. Just after Ben said "amen" after our
nightly prayer time, he squeezed my hand and said, "Praying with
you is the highlight of my day."

I can honestly say that the feeling is mutual. There is something
indescribably awesome—awesome in the true sense of the word—
about praying with the person you love most, the person with
whom you are in covenant with God, mandated by Him to be a
living picture of His Son's relationship with His Church. Don't get
me wrong; our prayers as married people don't get special treatment
and hover perpetually at the top of God's inbox (anyone seen *Bruce
Almighty?*). God hears and values all prayers equally, granted that
they are prayed with a repentant, obedient heart that harbors no
unforgiveness (see Psalm 66:18, Matthew 6:12, Proverbs 28:9,

and Mark 11:25). But when I pray with Ben, I feel safer, stronger, and absolutely unshakable. I feel like we are joining forces as two warriors marching across a battlefield, armed, dangerous, and oh so ready to simultaneously fight the armies of evil and obey the orders of our Commanding Officer.

God's Word has much to say about the importance and power of prayer. Here are just a few of the reasons why prayer is so significant and why it's crucial that every follower of Jesus has a dynamic prayer life:

* Prayer is the means by which we talk directly to our Creator (James 4:8)
* Prayer gives us the peace of God and guards our hearts (Philippians 4:6)
* Prayer supplies the answers to great mysteries (Jeremiah 33:3)
* When we don't know how to pray as we ought to, God's Holy Spirit intercedes (Romans 8:26)
* We can know without a doubt that when we pray for wisdom, we'll always receive it (James 1:5)
* It is God's will for us to pray continually (1 Thessalonians 5:17)
* If we ask anything in accordance with God's will, He hears us (1 John 5:14)

Ben and I haven't always considered prayer time the best time of our day. While we would pray together in the past, it was sporadic, and the prayers were often halfhearted and trite and felt rather laborious, to be completely honest. I had a feeling that if we weren't enjoying prayer, it was probable that God wasn't enjoying receiving them, as He likens prayers to incense rising into His nostrils ...and no one likes smelly incense.[39]

As God began to feel distant and our struggles stuck around, we knew we needed to make a change and get serious about prayer.

---

39 Psalm 141:2, Revelation 5:8

So we prioritized it. We persevered in our petitioning, even when it felt like we were hitting cement walls and that our prayers were getting no farther than the ceiling. We held each other accountable to lifting our requests to God and thanking Him for His goodness, even in late hours or when one of us was angry and by no means feeling spiritual or particularly grateful. And you know what? God honored our prayers, because now they were wholehearted. Now they were genuine and desperate for a touch from God. Now we were aware that without them, our marriage would be a pale, poor, and laughable imitation of Jesus' relationship with His bride, rather than a resplendent portrait that evokes curiosity and wonder from the world.

Are you and your spouse putting prayer first in your marriage? If not, I can tell you with the utmost certainty that it's time to humble yourself, perhaps in the following moments, and ask God to help you cherish and enjoy the gift of prayer as it ought to be. Then, despite a multitude of excuses and distractions that will try to tear you away from a time of stillness before Your King, pray anyway.

Take seriously the incredible privilege of talking with, crying to, and hearing from our Good Shepherd. Let Him lead you beside still waters. Allow Him to give you rest upon green pastures. Permit Him to give you the peace and confidence to endure any storm you and your spouse may face, from the stress of finances and burdens of life to the inevitable shadows of death. You will be amazed as your marriage transforms from a child's splatter-paint picture to a Michelangelo masterpiece, all through the power of prayer.

"There is no wonder more supernatural and divine in the life of a believer than the mystery and ministry of prayer...the hand of the child touching the arm of the Father and moving the wheel of the universe."

—A.B. Simpson

DAY 28

"Yell a loud no to the Devil and watch him scamper."

—James 4:7, MSG

While we were in my hometown for a wedding last weekend, my mom had me pull up YouTube on my laptop and type into the search bar, "small dog chases off two bears." You can imagine the dubious look I gave her. Was this video a Saturday Night Live skit, or perhaps an animated Pixar short? (My mom does love Pixar.) But, lo and behold, this 28-second video contained raw footage of a French bulldog chasing away two young bears from its owner's patio and garden in California. Ben and I watched in amazement. Then watched in amazement again.

Growing up on a small farm with at least five dogs at any given time, I know that a dog's size has nothing to do with its place within the canine pecking order. For example, during elementary and middle school, we had a ragtag pack of seven dogs, many of which were strays. Out of the seven, only two of them were smaller than the self-proclaimed "alpha dog," a female Blue Heeler named Sugar. The other four behaved as though she was, well, a full-grown

Grizzly. One look from her and they would all tuck their tails and stop in their tracks until she passed by.

As the name of her breed implies, Sugar the Blue Heeler inherently "heeled" the heifers and bulls on the farm, barking after them and nipping at their heels. And because she was the boss, she often heeled her fellow dogs as well, just to remind them of their place. (Luckily, she was more playful than aggressive with the other dogs; we never had to call on The Dog Whisperer!)

Watching the video of the bulldog and the bears, it dawned on me that this little dog's ferocity and boldness serve as a demonstration of how we are to be in the midst of spiritual attack.

The Bible describes Satan as a "roaring lion looking for someone to devour."[40] He isn't some bright red medieval-looking, long-tailed, pointy-eared imp holding a trident. He isn't just out to sit on your shoulder, whisper devious words, and cause a little mischief. Quite the contrary—he is like a *lion*, the chief of predators, on the prowl seeking to steal, kill, and destroy the human race.[41]

Like the bears in comparison to the French bull dog, and like Goliath in comparison to David, Satan is a giant, someone whom, with natural eyes, is terrifying and unbeatable. But, as the Word of God attests, he certainly *can* be beaten. As today's verse says, we have the authority to make him scamper away, just like the bears did when the bulldog went berserk on them.

Another translation of today's verse reads, "Resist the devil, and he will flee from you."[42] The Greek word for "resist" is *anthistémi*, and means "take a stand against," "hold one's ground," "forcefully declare one's personal conviction," "to keep one's possession," "ardently withstand without giving up."[43]

---

40   1 Peter 5:8, NIV
41   John 10:10
42   NIV
43   http://biblehub.com/greek/436.htm (accessed October 15, 2015)

PART 1: REFLECTIONS **69**

"Resist" is a pretty awesome word, right? When we view it through the lens of the original Greek text, we see that it is an active word of adamant stalwartness. Resisting doesn't mean we are dangling from a precipice, hanging on for dear life, begging our assailant to back off and leave us alone lest we crash onto the jagged rocks below. No, we are being forceful. We are declaring that the enemy has no right to steal from us or destroy any possession, whether physical, emotional, or otherwise. Like the French bulldog, we are "ardently withstanding," never backing down. In fact, we go on the offensive, effectively turning the tables on the devil, pursuing him in the name of Jesus so that he has no choice but to flee in abject terror at the Name above all names!

Whatever may sneak into your home today to steal your joy, destroy your hope, or kill your peace, don't hesitate to resist it passionately and fearfully in Jesus' name. No matter the size of the problem or person who is oppressing you, remember that God is bigger and infinitely greater. And if He is with you, as Paul rhetorically asks, who can be against you?[44]

> "It's not the size of the dog in the fight,
> it's the size of the fight in the dog."
>
> —Mark Twain

44 Romans 8:31

DAY 21

"Three things will last forever—faith, hope, and love—
and the greatest of these is love."

—1 Corinthians 13:13, NLT

We all know that verse. It's a favorite for Christian wedding ceremonies and home décor alike. As a lover of words, I pity the fact that our English language provides only one definition for the word "love," whereas the Greek gives four, each with distinctive meanings. They are:

- *Eros:* This word, not used in the New Testament, derived its name from the mythological Greek god of love, and refers to sexual love.
- *Storge:* This type of love describes the natural affection one has for his or her family members. In the New Testament, *storge* is used only twice, each time in its negative form, *astorgos*, which means "devoid of natural or instinctive affection, without affection to kindred."

* *Phileo:* Strong's Exhaustive Concordance defines this word as, "to be a friend to…fond of an individual or object; having affection for (as denoting attachment); a matter of sentiment or feeling." It describes close, warm, brotherly love, the kind that inspires friends to do nice things for one another.

* *Agapē:* This is the rendering of "love" we read in today's verse. It refers to a love that loves sacrificially. A love that loves the undeserving, even one's enemies. The kind of love that Christ displayed when He stretched out His arms on the cross and gave His sinless life for us. It is this type of love that the Bible says is the greatest.

Norman Geisler, in his book *Christian Ethics*, explained the nuances of each of the four words this way:

"Erotic love is egoistic. It says, 'My first and last consideration is myself.' Philic love is mutualistic. It says, 'I will give as long as I receive.' Agapic love, on the other hand, is altruistic, saying, 'I will give, requiring nothing in return.'"

As married people, we have likely felt and expressed all of the Greek iterations of love, and some more frequently than others. When we were just getting to know our significant other, we likely felt *phileo* love. The intensity of *phileo* increased so much that we knew we would be more than friends. We would be spouses, we would be lovers. That led to eros love, as we enjoyed our spouse intimately after the pastor said, "Man and wife" (at least, that's the order God intends). Next, as a small family, we experienced storge love.

It is *agapē* love that doesn't always come as naturally as the other three. In fact, it comes *supernaturally*, a testament to the presence of the Holy Spirit working in our hearts, helping us to love like Jesus. Indeed, we need this supernatural power from Almighty

God to turn the other cheek when someone strikes us, and to give our jacket also when someone sues us for a shirt.[45]

Jesus spoke about loving our enemies during His magnificent Sermon on the Mount:

> "If you love those who love you, what reward will you get? Are not even the tax collectors doing that? And if you greet only your own people, what are you doing more than others? Do not even pagans do that?"
>
> —*Matthew 5:46-47, NIV*

Why am I writing about *agapē* and loving our enemies when this is a *marriage* book? Because, again, going back to our marriage-loathing adversary, we must be on our guard against spiritual attacks, one of which is poisoning relationships with toxic feelings of hurt, bitterness, and anger. In other words, he wants to make husbands and wives enemies.

If you've been married long enough to unpack from your honeymoon, then you know what I mean. We've all gotten into squabbles, looked at our spouse, and had not-very-nice thoughts about them. Sometimes we have said those not-very-nice thoughts out loud, which got our spouse thinking and saying even worse things about us! Before you know it, we are enemies at war.

Like Jesus said in the passage above, the ungodly love those who love them. Why? Because it's natural to do so. We were born to respond favorably to kindness and to receive love without complaint. It doesn't require a regenerated heart. It is when we love the unlovable that we show the world, and the recipient of our love, that we have Holy Spirit-filled hearts, made new in Jesus Christ.

45 Matthew 5:39-40

Today, ask the Lord to help you live out the most important love of all, *agapē*. Before signs of a quarrel even begin to manifest between you and your spouse, ask Him to help you love like Jesus, not to retaliate with harshness, vitriol, or sarcasm. Each time you pray with your spouse, ask God to fill you both with sacrificial, unconditional, Christ-like love.

"There must be a stronger foundation than mere friendship or sexual attraction. Unconditional love, agapē love, will not be swayed by time or circumstances."

—*Stephen Kendrick*

DAY 22

"While he was eating, a woman came in with a beautiful alabaster jar of expensive perfume made from essence of nard. She broke open the jar and poured the perfume over his head."

—Mark 14:3, NLT

Today's verse comes from a memorable moment in the Gospels when Mary, one of Jesus' disciples, visits Him while He is dining at the house of Simon the leper (the *former* leper, that is) and shows her love for Him in a remarkable way.[46]

What Mary poured on Jesus's head wasn't some drug store brand of perfume. And it certainly didn't come in a plastic bottle. On the contrary, the container was made of alabaster, which is a hard, white, marble-looking stone, one used to build Solomon's famously beautiful temple.[47] In Song of Solomon, the man is described as having legs that are "pillars of alabaster."[48] In other

---

46 Simon is still called "the leper" to distinguish him from others named Simon, or Simeon, which was a common name among the Jews
47 1 Chronicles 29:2
48 Song of Solomon 5:15, NASB

words, this was a well revered rock! But it was the costly contents inside the jar that got the attention of those who witnessed her over-the-top act of love...

"Some of those at the table were indignant. 'Why waste such expensive perfume?' they asked. 'It could have been sold for a year's wages and the money given to the poor!' So they scolded her harshly."

—Mark 14:4-5, NLT

But Jesus was touched by what she had done. He called it a "good thing" and rebuked the others for criticizing her. He saw that, in her own beautiful and unique way, she was anointing His body for burial, as the time of His arrest and crucifixion was drawing closer.

Sure, the money from the perfume could have been used for a host of altruistic purposes. With it, she could have bought food and clothing for the needy or given it to Jesus to use as He saw fit. But only at that moment could she use it to bless her Lord and teacher, knowing His time on earth was growing short.

"'You will always have the poor among you, and you can help them whenever you want to. But you will not always have me,'" Jesus said to those who sneered (Mark 14:7, NLT).

Mary seemed to have a strong sense of what would please and bless Jesus most in the days leading up to His death. Anointing Him with what was inarguably one of her most expensive possessions sent the clear message to Him and the other disciples gathered there (as well as to you and me) that she loved Him with a deep, abiding, sacrificial *agapē* love, a love that poured out of her heart, just as the oil flowed out of the alabaster jar.

There's a wonderful Christian marriage book called *The 5 Love Languages* by Dr. Gary Chapman. In it, he identifies and outlines five ways ("languages") people show their love for others, as well as how they personally prefer to receive love. The languages are Words of Affirmation, Quality Time, Receiving Gifts, Acts of Service, and Physical Touch. In the story of Mary and her alabaster jar, we can deduce that one of her primary love languages was Acts of Service, and evidently—and not surprisingly!—Jesus spoke that language, too.

There is something to be learned from this story regarding loving others, particularly our spouse. The way we express love may not be the way our spouse best responds to love. For example, at the beginning of our marriage, I would give Ben little presents, because gift giving is one of my main love languages. Over the years, however, I've learned that the way to Ben's heart is actually via quality one-on-one time. I, on the other hand, appreciate words of affirmation and gifts, as I mentioned above. So rather than detailing my car to show his love for me (Ben's second primary love language is Acts of Service), Ben often buys me a bouquet of flowers, no special occasion necessary, and builds me up with encouraging, sometimes lovey-dovey words (which I love!).

How can you bless your spouse today? What will be the rare, aromatic oil that you pour over him or her? Whether it's planning a steak dinner at an upscale restaurant, or planting more hugs and kisses when you get home from work, take time to consider how you can speak the love language of your spouse. Then, ask God to help you become fluent in that language, even if it feels foreign to you. I promise that speaking each other's language will bring blessing to both of you as you grow and develop on multiple levels of intimacy.

> "You can always give without loving,
> but you can never love without giving."
>
> —Amy Carmichael

DAY 23

"Two people are better off than one, for they can help each other succeed. If one person falls, the other can reach out and help. But someone who falls alone is in real trouble."

—*Ecclesiastes 4:9-10, NLT*

This verse came to mind just last night as I was pushing through an especially tough workout at our gym. The workout looked simple on paper: seven rounds of 10 burpees, followed immediately by a 200-meter run…a *sprint*, if possible. Your score for the workout would be your slowest time out of the seven rounds, and you could rest as long as you wanted in between each. Easy peasy.

Not.

By the second round, I was already wondering how my husband could be so evil. After all, this particular workout was hatched in his brain. My lungs were burning. My legs, sore from the previous day's workout, were equally on fire. To make matters worse, the two giant dumpsters belonging to the Mexican restaurant adjacent to our gym were filled to the brim, emitting a stomach-churning potpourri.

I wanted to quit, and probably would have had it not been for my husband, who happened to be coaching that class, cheering me on.

"Think 'fast burpees.' Forget about the burpees. Just tune them out and get them done," he said. "Then go hard on the run."

By now, you're all too familiar with burpees and know that your mind can't exactly float merrily along in la la land while your body performs this powerhouse movement. However, by round five, I actually *was* able to tune them out…somewhat, at least. Because by then, Coach Ben was coaching our running, shouting at us, "Quick feet! You don't have to run fast, just move your feet in small, fast steps." (Perhaps he can explain the rationale behind this advice, because I associate "small, fast steps" with running, ha!) The general theme throughout each of his mini pep talks in between rounds seemed to be this: *Just keep moving.*

I normally don't do this until the workout is over, but I couldn't help myself… After round six, I bent over, lowered myself onto the floor, and lay down, thus assuming the official "I'm done-thank-goodness-that's-over" position in CrossFit.

After twenty seconds or so of my histrionics, Ben came over, and without a word, simply held out his hand. I knew I wasn't done yet, and so did he. Was I in pain? Yes. But was I in danger? No. Absolutely not. This workout was making me stronger, mentally and physically; stopping short would have been surrendering to it.

I know that last sentence might sound dramatic given the context of a silly workout, but it's true. Completing tough workouts translates powerfully into other facets of our lives. It gives us the confidence, strength, discipline, and determination we need to face the unpredictable obstacles life throws at us. But just like emotional and spiritual trials, physical trials often require more than our own internal motivation.

Today's verse tells us plainly that two are better than one. Destiny's Child and Kelly Clarkson might have sung the praises of independent women, and Willie Nelson might have been content with his Whiskey River, but the Word of God sings a different song, one which finds sweet harmony in man and woman working together.

Husbands and wives were made to be teammates. Made to love and respect, honor and cherish, encourage and care for each other. Without Ben's helping hand and motivating words, last night's workout would have left me in the dust. And it's no different when it comes to the tests I face outside the gym.

Without Ben, I have no doubt God would see me through life's valleys, but I know that with him, I have a tremendous advantage. I have someone who loves the Lord physically present to pick me up off the floor and cheer me on to the finish line. I have a best friend to pray beside, to go to war with, and rejoice with as conquerors in Christ. And that is a God-given gift that should never once be taken for granted.

"Coming together is a beginning; keeping together is progress; working together is success."

—*Henry Ford*

DAY 24

"'Therefore what God has joined together, let no one separate.'"

—Mark 10:9, NIV

A Barna study recently released some startling statistics about marriage. Those most pertinent for the purposes of this reflection are these: Thirty-two percent of all born again Christians have been divorced, as well as 26% of evangelical Christians.[49] Atheists have a divorce rate of 30% (that's two percent less than born again Christians, in case you missed that).

George Barna, director of the study, commented that it seems Americans have grown comfortable with divorce, viewing it as a natural part of life."

"There no longer seems to be much of a stigma attached to divorce; it is now seen as an unavoidable rite of passage," the researcher indicated. "Interviews with young adults suggest that they want their initial marriage to last, but are not particularly

49 https://www.barna.org/barna-update/article/15-familykids/42-new-marriage-and-divorce-statistics-released#.ViUR-_IViko (accessed October 19, 2015)

optimistic about that possibility. There is also evidence that many young people are moving toward embracing the idea of serial marriage, in which a person gets married two or three times, seeking a different partner for each phase of their adult life."[50]

That nearly one-third of "born again Christians" has been divorced is evidence of Satan's foothold in our marriages.

As I've stated elsewhere in this book, by dismantling God-ordained unions, the enemy not only cripples and embitters those who divorce, but also perpetuates the common secular perception that lifelong marriages are, at best, rarely achievable, and at worst, old fashioned and passé. This jaded mentality is undoubtedly responsible for the higher rates of cohabitation in which couples live together, even have children together, but avoid any serious commitment. If I weren't a follower of Christ, I'm convinced I too would share this prevalent, self-preserving philosophy. I'd likely ask, "Why say 'I do' when odds are good I'll say 'Nevermind, I don't' in just a few years time?"

Before I go on, I want to be clear that there are certainly legitimate grounds for divorce, such as unfaithfulness and ongoing abuse. But those two issues aside, too many couples today divorce willy-nilly. "We just grew apart" is perhaps one of the most recurring lines I read in the media regarding celebrity divorces, as well as, "It was a wonderful season in our lives, but we've moved on." Sometimes I catch myself reading between the lines. What they wanted to say was, "He made me happy for a while, but then just started irritating me." Or, "It was smooth sailing at the beginning, but after one storm too many, I abandoned ship."

We might expect such a casual regard for marriage from Hollywood. But among our Christian brothers and sisters, we

50 Ibid.

should observe a higher standard, one in which marriage is fought for as the sacred ordinance of joy, hope, and fulfillment that God created it to be. Sadly, however, we see that Christians' views on marriage have, for the most part, been weakened. If you want to get married, terrific. If you want to divorce, eh…as long as it makes you happy, go for it.

Malachi 2:16 says that God hates divorce. He knows the devastation it brings to those directly involved, as well as the damage it does to the picture of Christ and His bride that marriages are meant to project to the world. I believe God also hates divorce because He knows that by divorcing in the valley, we miss the glories of the mountaintop.

Throughout the scriptures, we see this pattern time and again: famine precedes abundance; valley precedes peak; mourning precedes joy. I've heard from multiple married couples, who have been together for decades, that the first 10 years were the hardest, but now they're more in love than they were on their wedding day! Many came close to calling it quits but are sure that because they didn't, God rewarded them generously for their perseverance and trust in Him to sustain them through thick and thin.

God never promised us an easy Christian life, let alone easy Christian married lives. What He *did* promise is that He will never leave us or forsake us.[51] Remember this when you feel you're at your wit's end and feel that the only way out is through the door marked, "divorce." That door is a mirage. It may look like a golden gateway into greener pastures, but in reality, it's a dead end, a lamentable barrier to the unimaginable blessings God has for you in your marriage.

51 Deuteronomy 31:6; Matthew 28:20

Meditate on the Lord's promises to bring you hope and a future, to work all things together for your good and to restore the years "that the swarming locusts have eaten."[52] Then trust Him to be faithful to those promises. And finally, rebuke and resist the devil (see Day 20) and tell him, in no uncertain terms, that he has no right to your marriage, your thoughts, or the thoughts of your spouse.

> "But as for me and my family, we will serve the Lord."
>
> —*Joshua 24:15, NLT*

---

52 Jeremiah 29:11; Romans 8:28; Joel 2:25

DAY 25

"Observe how the lilies of the field grow"

—*Matthew 6:28, NASB*

If there's one word I could use to describe how the majority of Americans feel today, it's "busy." Between time spent doing household chores, working a full-time job, taking care of kids, and trying to balance extracurricular activities and a social life, many men and women are stretched thin, feeling burnt out and worn out at the end of every day. But why? What are we working so hard for?

Sure, we rightly want to provide for our families. The Bible instructs us to do so.[53] But I think that many young working couples today keep so painfully busy for other reasons as well: to accumulate more stuff, keep up with Joneses, take more trips, and in some ways, increase their sense of self-worth.

I love these words of Jesus':

"For this reason I say to you, do not be worried about your life, as to what you will eat or what you will drink; nor for your body, as to what you will put on. Is not life more than food, and the body more than clothing? Look at the birds of the air, that they do not sow, nor reap nor gather into barns, and yet your heavenly Father feeds them. Are you not worth much more than they?"

—Matthew 6:25-16, NASB

Think about our culture and what it values most. If you're at a loss for ideas, just turn on your TV or go to Facebook for two minutes. You will quickly see that we are obsessed with our *selves*, with indulging ourselves, comforting ourselves, treating ourselves, and defending ourselves, even if our actions fly in the face of biblical teaching. And because we strive to satisfy Self, we are constantly thinking about material things with which to pamper it, such as food and clothing, just like Jesus said.

But striving is unending. Once we have as much as the Joneses, we'll find another person or group of people to emulate. Once we travel to all the trendy vacation hotspots where our friends (or Facebook pseudo-friends) have been, we'll make plans and start saving for the next dream getaway. Once we get that promotion we've been working so hard for, we'll set our eyes on the next rung of the ladder and proceed to climb into the empty clouds of our own ambition.

Eventually, striving is also exhausting. We can sustain the cycle of setting and achieving goals that feed our flesh and stroke our egos for years, perhaps decades, but in the end, as King Solomon wrote, it's all vanity.[54] "What do people get for all their hard work under the sun?" he wrote.[55]

Like the Egyptian pharaohs who prepared for their underworld

54 Ecclesiastes 1:2
55 Ecclesiastes 1:3

journey by equipping their tombs with food, amulets, jewelry, pets, and even small statues symbolizing servants, we in the 21st century seem to be hoarding possessions like they'll be going with us into heaven. Of course, we know this isn't true, but our actions, by and large, indicate otherwise. We allow the world to sweep us into its fast-paced current in which busyness and stress are somehow glorified and rest and peace are viewed as weak, mundane, and unexciting.

I love this poem by Elizabeth Cheney, titled "The Robin and the Sparrow":

> *Said the robin to the sparrow,*
>   *"I should really like to know,*
> *Why these anxious human beings*
>   *Rush about and worry so."*
> *Said the sparrow to the robin,*
>   *"Friend I think that it must be,*
> *That they have no Heavenly Father,*
>   *Such as cares for you and me."*

You may not hear this every day, but I implore you to think like a bird. Think like a lily. These and thousands of other creatures know instinctively that they are in the all-knowing mind, all-seeing eyes, and all-caring hands of their Heavenly Father. Their work brings honor to Him, not to themselves. All that they own—feathers, petals, food, nests…—are cherished not as trophies they have earned, but as gifts they have graciously been given. As such, they seek to be faithful stewards, greeting each morning with a heart eager to magnify their Maker, and welcoming each night with a soul thankful for another day's provision.

"Riches have never yet given anybody either peace or rest."

—*Billy Sunday*

DAY 26

For in six days the LORD made the heavens, the earth, the sea,
and everything in them; but on the seventh day he rested. That is
why the LORD blessed the Sabbath day and set it apart as holy."

—Exodus 20:11, NLT

We're all familiar with the creation story in Genesis. In a
theological nutshell, God made the world in six days and rested
on the seventh (Genesis 2:2). Please understand, God was not
worn out! He simply rested from His work to establish the pattern
which mankind would later follow. The corresponding law was
given 2,500 years after creation to Moses on Mount Sinai (Exodus
20:11). It was given not only so the Israelites would reflect on the
perfect state of creation and man's relationship with God before
sin crept in, but also so they would remember their deliverance
from the bonds of Egypt:

> "Remember that you were slaves in Egypt and that the Lord
> your God brought you out of there with a mighty hand and an
> outstretched arm. Therefore the Lord your God has commanded
> you to observe the Sabbath day."[56]
>
> —*Deuteronomy 5:15*

As with the Old Covenant sacrifices and ceremonies recorded in the Old Testament, the Sabbath was a picture of something far greater that was to come; it was a precursor to the rest we find in Messiah. The Sabbath is no longer about a religious doctrine to be strictly upheld with tedious rules and rituals and enforced with severe punishment. It is about abiding in the eternal rest provided by Jesus Christ who came to "fulfill" the law (Matt. 5:17).

Paul wrote: *"Therefore do not let anyone judge you by what you eat or drink, or with regard to a religious festival, a New Moon celebration or a Sabbath day. These are a shadow of the things that were to come; the reality, however, is found in Christ."* —*Colossians 2:16-17*

You're perhaps wondering how the Old Covenant law of the Sabbath and its emphasis on rest applies to you. Let me tell you! Just as the dietary laws found in the Old Testament were not randomly formulated by our Creator, neither was His notion of an entire day devoted purely to rest.[57]

In the good ol' days, Sundays were set apart in America as a day to rest from work, gather for worship, and enjoy time with family and friends. My mom grew up in the '50s and '60s and can't recall a single restaurant, gas station, or department store ever being open for business on Sunday! My grandmother would cook a lavish Sunday brunch and invite the whole family over

---

56 The Hebrew word for Sabbath is *Shabbat* which means "to rest or to lay aside labor." Every seventh day of the week, *Shabbat* was to be set apart as a day of rest for God's people. Jesus taught, "'The Sabbath was made for man, and not man for the Sabbath'" (Mark 2:27).
57 Check out my book *Fit for Faith* for more on the "why" behind the Bible's dietary laws.

after church. They'd spend the entire day simply eating good food, laughing at jokes, sharing stories, and kicking back. My, how times have changed.

Today, Sunday is just an extension of Saturday. Many kids have sporting events on Sundays, teenagers go to the mall and out to eat with friends, countless college kids nurse hangovers and celebrate one more day of weekend, and adults often go in to the office to catch up on paperwork or get a head start on the work week. The concept of rest seems to have become a luxury to be indulged once in a blue moon, not a necessity to enjoy every week.

Rest is important for everything in creation. Here are a few examples:

* Land that is continually worked without being given rest or replenished becomes infertile.
* If music didn't have spaces of silences and rest, we would only hear noise.
* If our hearts didn't rest between beats, they would stop.
* If various species of animals did not sleep at night, they would get eaten instead.
* If some animals didn't hibernate, they would freeze or starve to death.

Any physician will tell you that rest is essential for good health. When we're deprived of adequate sleep, we put ourselves at risk for sickness and other side effects such as difficulty concentrating, poor mood, and trouble remembering and thinking clearly. And as fit men and women, we can negate all the hard work we did in the gym and increase our risks for injury by forgoing much needed rest.

When I was anorexic, I stubbornly went against the advice of my trainer and worked out for at least an hour, seven days a week.[58] I reasoned I could burn more calories by not taking a day off. Of course, it is true that we do burn calories by working out all seven days, but our bodies become less efficient at recovering and rebuilding when we overwork them. I was, undeniably, "overtraining."

Overtraining occurs when a person ignores the body's need to rest, forcing the muscles to remain in a state of damage because they aren't given enough time to repair. Along with my poor diet, overtraining contributed to my constant feeling of lethargy and weakness.

After I became healthy again, I immediately felt recharged and refreshed each time I stepped into the gym after a day of unadulterated rest. Think of your body as a cell phone; putting it on the charger for a few seconds when the battery is almost dead won't give it very much juice. Likewise, our bodies need ample rest to be totally rejuvenated.

A day should be set aside not only to rest our bodies, but our souls as well. God said through the prophet Isaiah:

> "If you keep your feet from breaking the Sabbath and from doing as you please on my holy day, if you call the Sabbath a delight and the LORD's holy day honorable, and if you honor it by not going your own way and not doing as you please or speaking idle words, then you will find your joy in the LORD, and I will cause you to ride on the heights of the land and to feast on the inheritance of your father Jacob.
>
> —Isaiah 58:13-14

I believe this passage reflects the true nature of God's heart for the Sabbath. God desires that we honor Him with one of our most

---

58 To read more about my struggle with anorexia and exercise bulimia, check out my memoir, Immeasurable: Diving into the Depths of God's Love.

precious possessions—our time. I fear too many Christians go their "own way" and "speak idle words" every day of the week, never distinguishing a "holy day," whether Sunday or another day, to spend with their Creator and Lord. We make our own plans, stay busy, chitchat, go here, go there, keep the TV on, the stereo playing, smartphone apps running, seldom calling the Sabbath—the laying aside of work—"a delight" or "honorable."

God says that if we draw near to Him, He will draw near to us (James 4:8). The above verse from Isaiah tells us if we honor a Sabbath day, we will find our joy in the Lord. God isn't going to descend into our living room one day a week, take us by the hand, and guide us into a quiet room for some one-on-one time. And we can't leave it up to our preachers to flip on the "Sabbath switch" for 30 minutes a week inside a sanctuary. God longs for us to come to Him personally!

> "But when you pray, go into your room, close the door
> and pray to your Father, who is unseen. Then your Father,
> who sees what is done in secret, will reward you."
>
> *—Matthew 6:6*

It's up to us to come to Him for fellowship. God has given us the awesome privilege of entering into His presence, but we must be willing to open the door.

This day of rest is to be a time of physical, spiritual, emotional, and mental renewal. Let's let Jesus be our example. Jesus spent His Saturdays, the Jewish Sabbath day, delighting in God's Word, teaching others, healing the sick, freeing the demonized. He shows us that the Sabbath is no longer a dreaded law to uphold, but a joyful day to embrace!

Resting from our work, our studies, our obligations, and our workout routines is a God-ordained command given to enrich every fiber of our being. With no time limits, no scheduled appointments, and no pressures, all we're left with is the amazing rest that comes from communing with our Creator.

> "Truly my soul waiteth upon God: from him cometh my salvation. He only is my rock and my salvation; he is my defense; I shall not be greatly moved."
>
> —*Psalm 61:1-2*

DAY 27

"Taste and see that the LORD is good;
blessed is the one who takes refuge in him."

—*Psalm 34:8*

Have you ever been at a fancy restaurant, whose menu has more foreign words than English ones, and gone out on a limb by ordering something completely new to you? And when you reluctantly put the exotic morsel on your tongue, were you blown away by how delicious it was and wondered where it had been all your life?

Perhaps you're not the adventurous type when it comes to food, so, like me, you stick to the basics—no duck liver or pork cheeks, thank you very much! But maybe your spouse, your daring other half, is one who orders those avant-garde, off-the-wall dishes. Ben is this way. He had extra opportunities to be this way while we were on our honeymoon on the beautiful Caribbean island of Saint Lucia. Each time we dined at the resort's restaurant, or the hotel across the street famous for infusing every entrée and appetizer with chocolate, he would choose something out of the ordinary, like Cacao Beer Jerked Chicken or Plantain Gratin with Coconut

Rum Sauce. And every time, his eyes would light up upon the first taste, and then these words would erupt from his lips:

"You have to try this!"

No matter how hard I resisted or how much I insisted that he should have his newfound favorite food all to himself, he wouldn't relent. He would hold a forkful in front of me until I gave in and agreed to taste and see that his meal was good. I was always glad I did!

We are like this in other ways outside of food, too. For example, if I see a good movie that I really love, I'll blast Twitter and Facebook with my enthusiastic praise of it (I did this most recently with War Room. Have you seen it yet?!). If Ben, a self-professed nerd, learns of a productivity app for my phone that he knows will help me stay on task during the day, he will email me immediately and tell me about it. When we love someone, we want to bless him or her with gifts that will delight, encourage, and assist them. This is how God is with us.

Today's verse comes from a man, King David, who had personally tasted of God's goodness and, led of the Holy Spirit, encouraged the people of Israel—and all God's people, indirectly—to partake of the divine Bread of Life. He didn't want to keep the sweet-tasting, life-changing good news of God's grace and faithfulness to himself. He didn't want people to merely hear about it, but to *experience* it.

I wonder how many of us need to stop simply watching other Christians receive and enjoy the Lord's goodness and have a taste ourselves. How many of us need to step out of our comfort zones and embrace with open arms the precious promises of His Word? How many of us need to trust God, even when doing so goes against our instincts and worldly wisdom?

Today with your spouse, examine your hearts to see if there is any area in your life together that hasn't been fully surrendered to the Lord. What fears are you holding onto? What unforgiveness are you harboring? What doubts are you giving in to? What past disappointments and failures are polluting your soul with feelings of unworthiness and hopelessness?

Whatever the situation may be, consider the Bible your blueprint for moving onward and upward. Don't study it like a dry historical text, but treasure it as God's love letter to you, filled with His promises to deliver you, restore you, comfort you, and provide for you. Come to it each night like a grand banquet to be savored. Taste and see that the Lord is good!

"Faith is not belief without proof, but trust without reservation."

—D. Elton Trueblood

DAY 28

" ... put a knife to your throat if you are given to gluttony."

—*Proverbs 23:2, NIV*

Before I begin, I wish to ease any concerns about the violent nature of today's verse. According to the Jamieson-Fausset-Brown Bible Commentary, the phrase "put a knife to your throat" is an Eastern expression that can be interpreted to mean "put a restraint on your appetite." With that said, let's continue, knowing that if our self-control ever slips at the dinner table, we can live to see another meal!

According to a 2012 Gallup poll, 27.2 percent of Americans are obese, and 35.5 percent overweight.[59] These figures probably come as no surprise to you considering the pleasure-crazed, five-senses-satisfying society in which we live. A short drive down the street will take you past (or straight to!) fast food restaurants whose aim it is tempt your taste buds with mouth-watering burgers and crispy

59 http://www.gallup.com/poll/165671/obesity-rate-climbing-2013.aspx
    (accessed October 22, 2015)

super-sized servings of fries. A night at the movies often makes buckets of popcorn and liters of soda the main attraction. Birthday parties and holiday feasts boast platters and platefuls of casseroles, cookies, chips and dips to make merrier our celebration. We often find ourselves eating not because we are hungry, but because we experience fleeting moments of pleasure bursting from the flavors of our favorite foods. When those moments vanish, we're on to the next bite, then the next bite…

According to the Merriam-Webster dictionary, "gluttony" is defined as "excess in eating or drinking." Having a slice of cake on our birthdays or enjoying a box of candy at the theater isn't gluttony. It's when the act of eating becomes excessive and all-consuming that it becomes gluttonous.

Unfortunately, we live in a culture that makes it all too easy, all too acceptable, to nibble to our heart's content. We're encouraged by family members to go back for seconds, urged by advertisements to get the combo meal and super-size it. Rarely do people call our overeating to our attention, and so the notion that it is sinful and selfish tends to elude us.

Sins can be readily identified with a simple question: Will doing this eventually harm me or someone else? From cigarette smoking to lusting, from cheating on a test to cheating on your spouse, every sin carries with it a harmful repercussion if we don't repent and turn back onto the narrow road. Smoking may lead to larynx or lung cancer, lusting to a pornography addiction and damaged relationships, and so forth. Gluttony sows seeds of obesity, which when watered consistently grow into fearsome, health-choking blossoms of diabetes, heart disease, and cancer. In short, it puts a knife to its partaker's throat.

Don't be a slave to your appetite. Instead, strive to be a steward of the marvelous, masterfully designed body God's given you. You honor Him when you honor your temple with moderation and discipline. You show love for your spouse when you lovingly nourish your body, and you serve as a beneficial, even life-saving, example to others.

"Self-control is the exercise of inner strength under the direction of sound judgement that enables us to do, think, and say the things that are pleasing to God."

—*Jerry Bridges*

DAY 29

"I know that my redeemer lives and that
in the end he will stand upon the earth"

—*Job 19:25, NIV*

Job loved the Lord and had been abundantly blessed with a large family, land, and extraordinary affluence; the dude owned seven-thousand sheep, three-thousand camels, five-hundred yoke of oxen, and five-hundred donkeys. Job 1:3 says he was "the greatest man among all the people of the East."

You've probably heard his story:

Satan—literally, the "Adversary"—is allowed by God Himself to torment Job. This ages-old "Accuser" believes Job will curse God when his health, wealth, and family are destroyed. Despite losing his possessions seemingly overnight—including all 10 of his children—and suffering painful boils from head to toe, Job continues to worship and trust God:

"Naked I came out of my mother's womb, and naked shall I return:
the Lord has given, and the Lord has taken away;
blessed be the name of Lord."
—Job 1:20-21, ESV

That's not to say Job didn't cry out in his distress or ask God for reprieve, for just a moment's glimmer in an hour of gloom. In fact, many times Job could not perceive God's presence at all! But Job's faith was so firmly fixed, his spirit so unshakeable, that not one sinful, murmuring word of cursing or complaint ever escaped his lips. He humbly acquiesced to what God had ordained and endured the depths of this world's sorrows with a spirit fully surrendered to following the Father, despite the bleak horizon. After all, he didn't know how his story would end…

The story did end very happily for Job. His health returned, and his wealth was restored with double the number of livestock, seven more sons and three more daughters! (His original 10 kids were in Heaven, alive and well!)

But what if Job's story hadn't ended so well? What if he'd died a lonely, diseased, childless widower without a penny to his name? He didn't know all along throughout his suffering that the tide would turn in his favor and that all would be restored. He only knew that the Lord was alive and reigning on His throne. And that was enough.

Is that enough for you?

Today, ask yourself how you might respond if everything you worked for and everyone you loved, including your spouse, was stripped away. Would you do as Job's wife urged him to do and curse the Lord? Would you become ravaged with guilt and fear, worrying that you'd somehow offended Almighty God? Or would you, like Job, remain faithful, deriving all the strength you need from the simple yet mind-blowing fact that your Redeemer lives, He is Lord of lords, and all things are in subjection under his feet, even the work of the devil (Ephesians 1:22)?

Jesus says it best:

"I have told you these things, so that in me you may have peace. In this world you will have trouble. But take heart! I have overcome the world."

—John 16:33 (NIV)

The greatest Treasure you will ever have can never be taken away. Let Him be enough for you every hour of every day.

DAY 30

"Now one of them, when he saw that he had been healed,
turned back, glorifying God with a loud voice"

—Luke 17:15, NASB

Jesus had just healed 10 lepers who had desperately called out to Him for mercy. As long as they had leprosy, they were considered outcasts due to the highly contagious nature of their disease. Jesus, this benevolent rabbi and amazing miracle worker they'd heard much about, was their only hope for returning to a normal life. Without hesitation, Jesus answered their request by sending them to the priests so they could declare the men cleansed and cleared for interaction with the rest of society.

His healing power was already manifesting within their broken bodies. Their prayers had been answered. They were experiencing the grace and omnipotence of the Living God first hand; because of Him, they would be among their friends and embracing their families in a matter of hours.

Apparently, thoughts of home and a return to normal life were all that filled the minds of nine of the 10 men healed that day in the lepers' village. Only one, when he noticed the healing overtaking his flesh, turned around and went back to Jesus where he fell on his face in a beautiful posture of thanksgiving.

How often are we like the nine former lepers? How often do we cry out to God for a sign, a miracle, a break, or a breakthrough only to neglect giving thanks when our prayers are answered? We receive the answer or blessing we've long desired, yet don't take the time to lift our hands and open our mouths in thanks to the One Who sent it.

We live in a world that glorifies independence and self-sufficient, self-empowered, "self-made" men and women. We're told that we can endure and achieve anything if we just put our minds to it, set goals, and give our all. But the truth is, we aren't self-sufficient. Whether we acknowledge it or not, every open door, every good and perfect gift, comes from above, not from within.[60]

But oh the blessing and joy that follow when we fall at the feet of the Giver of all good gifts! Our gratitude draws us closer to Him as we think upon His faithfulness and remember that we would be sin-covered outcasts begging outside His kingdom's gates without the ultimate gift He gave on the cross 2,000 years ago.

Today, set aside time with your spouse to go to Jesus with humility in your heart and thanks on your lips. Whether it's a miraculous healing, a smooth and successful job interview, a resolved bone of contention between you and your mate, or merely a sunny, stress-free afternoon, we have much to be thankful for.

"Be thankful in all circumstances, for this is God's will for you who belong to Christ Jesus."

—1 Thessalonians 5:18, NLT

---

60 James 1:17

DAY 31

"And do not forget to do good and to share with others,
for with such sacrifices God is pleased"

—Hebrews 13:16, NIV

I don't know about you, but in my life, "doing good," as today's verse instructs, isn't too hard to forget. For example, at the grocery store recently, I spotted an elderly woman having a difficult time pulling a shopping cart out of its row. I didn't think twice about going over and yanking it free for her. And when it was apparent that a family at the airport recently was running late for their flight, I remembered to "do good" and insist they pass in front of me in the security line. My mama didn't raise no ill-mannered fool!

What doesn't come so easily to me is the "to share" part of today's Scripture. In each of the occurrences above, I hardly spoke. A shy and introverted person by nature, I'm not one to strike up conversation with distressed grandmothers at the store or stressed-out families on the go. I'm not one who likes to share with strangers.

But sharing is a major calling and responsibility for us as

Christians. How else is the Gospel and God's love made known to the world but through sharing? How else do we let others know how Christ has saved, set free, and transformed us but through opening our mouths, pulling out our pens, or firing up our computers to reach hurting, wandering souls? It is only when we exit our cozy turtle shells, forget restrictive adjectives and labels like "timid," "introverted" and "loner," and allow the Holy Spirit to direct our steps and inspire our words that God's Kingdom work can be accomplished through us.

Now, I'm not saying that we must quote John 3:16 to every cashier, courtesy clerk, and cab driver we encounter; however, based on God's Word, we must not be opposed to or intimidated by such opportunities. If you feel God directing you to dialogue with someone whose day needs brightening, whose hope needs stirring, whose heart needs softening, trust that the Lord will give you the words to say and bring to your remembrance the things His Son has told you in Scripture (John 14:26).

No matter how uncomfortable it may make us to ask a stranger if we can pray for them or to invite a mere acquaintance to church, we must remember that it is Christ in us who is truly doing the work. He is the one knocking at the heart's door of those we share Him with. We should be glad and grateful to announce His visit, knowing that the sacrifice of our time and the escape from our comfort zones pleases our Lord and Savior.

Who can you and your spouse reach out to today? How can you show that person, or persons, the love and hope of Jesus Christ? What lessons from your own journey of faith can you share with them? How can you use your marriage as a platform from which to proclaim God's faithfulness?

"Let others report bad news; we'll share the good news."

—*Woodrow Kroll*

PART II
PARTNER
WORKOUTS

IMPORTANT: *Be sure to take time (5 to 10 minutes) to* **stretch** *at the end of every workout, focusing on the muscles most emphasized that day, as well as any areas that feel particularly tight or sore.*

Stretching improves circulation, increases flexibility, helps maximize the range of motion in your joints, and reduces soreness and stress! Each stretch should be held between **15 and 30 seconds** *and should feel good. If it becomes painful, ease up a bit, breathe deep, and go slower.*

You will find the recommended stretches and their descriptions in the Appendix following the main exercises.

Also essential to any workout, no matter what it is, is a proper warmup.

WHY WARM UP?

Because warming up properly is full of benefits, including:

- Elevation of body temperature
- Increase blood flow in the muscles
- Improves efficient cooling
- Improves range of motion
- Reduces incidence and likelihood of musculoskeletal injuries
- Supplies adequate blood flow to heart
- Provides rehearsal of movements performed in the workout
- Mental preparation

As you can see, the warm-up prepares us for an effective and rewarding workout. When the workout (the fun part!) begins, our blood is flowing hot, our hearts are pumping strong, and our minds are thinking fast, each part of us giving one-hundred percent to the exercises at hand.

In other words: ***Don't Skip the Warm-Up!***

DAY 1 WORKOUT

WARM-UP

- [ ] 30 walking lunges with twist over lunging knee (15 each leg)
- [ ] 30 air squats
- [ ] 10 walk-out/walk-ins
- [ ] 30 jumping jacks
- [ ] 15 jump squats
- [ ] 400-meter run (0.25 miles)[61]

WORKOUT

Set a timer for 15 minutes and perform as many rounds as you can of the following circuit:

- [ ] 10 partner push-ups with reach
- [ ] 10 jump squats, alternating with your partner each rep
- [ ] 20 stationary lunges, alternating with your partner each rep
- [ ] 10 right side plank hip dips, alternating with your partner each rep
- [ ] 10 left side plank hip dips, alternating with your partner each rep

---

61 If doing the WODs at home, I recommend going outside (as long as it's safe!) and approximating this distance. If you're at the gym, hop on the treadmill!

DAY 2 WORKOUT

WARM-UP

2 rounds:

- ☐ 30 butt kicks (10 each leg)
- ☐ 20 high kicks (10 each leg)
- ☐ 20 mountain-climbers (right/left is 1 rep)
- ☐ 10 slow air squats (lower for 5 seconds)
- ☐ 5 burpees

WORKOUT

This workout is relay style, meaning one of you will go first on each exercise and rest as the other completes it. The starting partner may not start subsequent exercises until the second partner is done with his or her exercise.

Time yourselves as you complete the following as fast as you can with proper form:

- ☐ 400-meter run (0.25 miles on the treadmill)
- ☐ 20 burpees
- ☐ 400-meter run (0.25 miles on the treadmill)
- ☐ 15 burpees
- ☐ 400-meter run (0.25 miles on the treadmill)
- ☐ 10 burpees

DAY 3 WORKOUT

WARM-UP

- [ ] 20 world's greatest stretch (10 each side)
- [ ] 20 jumping jacks
- [ ] 20 scorpions
- [ ] 20 iron crosses
- [ ] 20 high knees
- [ ] 10 mountain-climbers (right/left is 1 rep)

WORKOUT

Set a timer and perform the following as fast as you can, using proper form, of course! Only one partner works at a time; the other partner rests until it's his or her turn. Each partner must complete the given number of repetitions.

5 rounds:

- [ ] 10 Superman
- [ ] 20 scissor jumps (each side counts as a rep)
- [ ] 30 bicycle crunches (each side counts as a rep)

DAY 4—REST DAY

DAY 5 WORKOUT

WARM-UP

- [ ] 400-meter jog (0.25 miles on treadmill)
- [ ] 10 walk-out/walk-ins
- [ ] 20 arm circles each direction
- [ ] 20 walking lunges with twist over the lunging knee
- [ ] 20 air squats
- [ ] 10 burpees

WORKOUT

Set a timer for 18 minutes and perform as many rounds as you can of the following circuit:

- [ ] 10 partner push-ups with shoulder tap
- [ ] 10 scissor jumps, alternating with your partner each rep
- [ ] 20 reverse stationary lunges, alternating with your partner each rep
- [ ] 20 partner sit-ups, alternating with your partner each rep (If you don't have an AbMat, place a pillow or rolled-up towel above your waistband to help support your lower back.)

DAY 6 WORKOUT

WARM-UP

- [ ] 400-meter jog (0.25 miles on treadmill)
- [ ] 20 lunges, holding at the bottom for 3 seconds each rep
- [ ] 40 butt kicks
- [ ] 40 high knees
- [ ] 20 high kicks
- [ ] 60-second plank hold
- [ ] 30-second plank hold, right side
- [ ] 30-second plank hold, left side

WORKOUT

This workout is relay style, meaning one of you will go first on each exercise and rest as the other completes it. The starting partner may not start subsequent exercises until the second partner is done with his or her exercise.

Time yourselves as you complete the following four times through:

- [ ] 200-meter run (0.12 miles on treadmill)
- [ ] 15 reptiles
- [ ] 30 Russian twists
- [ ] 45 jumping jacks

DAY 7 WORKOUT

WARM-UP

- [ ] 50 jumping jacks
- [ ] 200-meter jog (0.12 miles on treadmill)
- [ ] 20 butt kicks
- [ ] 20 high knees
- [ ] 20 high kicks
- [ ] 20 lateral lunges (10 each leg)
- [ ] 20 wall push-ups
- [ ] 20 arm circles each direction

BENCHMARK WORKOUT

*Record your scores for each section of this workout; you will be doing this workout again and can look at them later and see how you've improved!

Complete the following with your spouse in the order given, with proper form:

- [ ] 800-meter run as fast as you can (0.5 miles on treadmill)
- [ ] Rest 2 minutes.
- [ ] 2 minutes of as many air squats as possible
- [ ] Rest 1 minute.
- [ ] 2 minutes of as many push-ups as possible
- [ ] Rest 1 minute.
- [ ] 2 minutes of as many pendulum lunges as possible

DAY 8—REST DAY

DAY 9 WORKOUT

WARM-UP

- [ ] 800-meter jog (0.5 miles)
- [ ] 10 walk-out/walk-ins
- [ ] 20 scorpions
- [ ] 20 iron crosses
- [ ] 20 sit-ups (If you don't have an AbMat, place a pillow or rolled-up towel above your waistband to help support your lower back.)
- [ ] 10 air squats
- [ ] 10 jump squats

WORKOUT

Time yourselves as you complete the following six times through:

- [ ] 10 partner burpees
- [ ] 20 one-legged Romanian deadlifts (10 each leg; perform these simultaneously with your partner)
- [ ] 10 plank-and-jumps each partner (switch spots after 10 reps)

DAY 18 WORKOUT

WARM-UP

- [ ] 400-meter jog
- [ ] 30 mock kettlebell swings
- [ ] 20 walking lunges with twist over lunging knee
- [ ] 10 slow air squats (lower for 5 seconds, and hold at the bottom for 5 seconds)
- [ ] 60-second plank hold
- [ ] 30-second plank hold, right side
- [ ] 30-second plank hold, left side

WORKOUT

Set a timer for 20 minutes and perform as many rounds as you can of the following circuit. Only one partner works at a time; the other partner rests until it's his or her turn. Each partner must complete the given number of repetitions.

- [ ] 10 lateral lunges (5 each leg)
- [ ] 10 knee-tucks
- [ ] 20 squat pulses
- [ ] 20 bicycle crunches

DAY 11 WORKOUT

WARM-UP

- [ ] 400-meter jog (0.25 miles on treadmill)
- [ ] 20 walking lunges
- [ ] 20 wall push-ups
- [ ] 20 arm circles each direction

3 rounds:

- [ ] 20 butt kicks
- [ ] 20 high knees
- [ ] 10 high kicks
- [ ] 20 jumping jacks
- [ ] 10 reptiles

WORKOUT

This workout is relay style, meaning one of you will go first on each exercise and rest as the other completes it. The starting partner may not start subsequent exercises until the second partner is done with his or her exercise.

Time yourselves as you complete the following as fast as you can with proper form:

- [ ] 200-meter run (0.12 miles on treadmill)
- [ ] 20 one-legged deadlifts with one-legged hop (10 reps each side)
- [ ] 10 mountain-climbers
- [ ] 400-meter run (0.25 miles on treadmill)
- [ ] 18 one-legged deadlifts with one-legged hop (9 reps each side)

☐ 10 mountain-climbers

☐ 800-meter run (0.5 miles on treadmill)

☐ 16 one-legged deadlifts with one-legged hop (8 reps each side)

☐ 10 mountain-climbers

DAY 12—REST DAY

The workouts from here on out will include equipment to help you take the intensity up a notch! Please refer to the Prologue for a list of recommended home gym equipment. Note that the only mandatory equipment is a pair of dumbbells and a kettlebell.

DAY 13 WORKOUT

WARM-UP

- [ ] 400-meter jog (0.25 miles on treadmill)
- [ ] 30 mock kettlebell swings
- [ ] 30 jumping jacks
- [ ] 20 arm circles each direction
- [ ] 20 wall push-ups
- [ ] 10 push-ups

WORKOUT

The first partner will perform the first set of reps, followed by the second partner. When Partner 2 is done, Partner 1 will start on the kettlebell swings.

10-9-8-7-6-5-4-3-2-1 reps alternating between:

- [ ] dumbbell push-press
- [ ] Russian kettlebell swings

After you finish this, each of you take turns holding a plank as long as you can for three sets.

DAY 14 WORKOUT

WARM-UP

3 rounds:

- ☐ 20 reverse lunges (10 each leg)
- ☐ 5 walk-out/walk-ins
- ☐ 10 air squats
- ☐ 10 push-ups

WORKOUT

Complete, with proper form, 30-24-18-12-6 reps of the workout below, dividing the repetitions between the two of you however you wish. Only one partner works at a time. For example, Partner 1 can do 15 reps of the first exercise, then rest as Partner 2 does 15 reps. Alternately, Partner 1 can do 10 reps, then rest as Partner 2 does 10 reps, or 15 reps, depending on his or her preference. Partner 1 would then resume the sumo deadlift high pulls to complete five more reps.

- ☐ sumo deadlift high pulls with kettlebell
- ☐ Russian twists holding kettlebell (each side is one rep)
- ☐ jump squats

DAY 15 WORKOUT

WARM-UP

- [ ] 200-meter jog (0.12 miles on treadmill)
- [ ] 30 jumping jacks
- [ ] 30 mock kettlebell swings
- [ ] 20 lunges with 3-second hold at the bottom
- [ ] 20 iron crosses
- [ ] 20 good-mornings
- [ ] 10 burpees

WORKOUT

Time yourselves as you complete the workout below seven times through. Partners work simultaneously. Each partner must complete the given number of reps, and both should be done with one exercise before moving on to the next.

- [ ] 10 renegade rows (5 each arm)
- [ ] 12 suitcase deadlifts with dumbbells
- [ ] 200-meter run (0.12 miles on treadmill)

DAY 16—REST DAY

DAY 17 WORKOUT

WARM-UP

- [ ] 50 jumping jacks
- [ ] 200-meter jog (0.12 miles on treadmill)
- [ ] 20 butt kicks
- [ ] 20 high knees
- [ ] 20 high kicks
- [ ] 20 lateral lunges (10 each leg)
- [ ] 20 wall push-ups
- [ ] 20 arm circles each direction

BENCHMARK WORKOUT

*Record your scores for each section of this workout; you will be doing this workout again and can also refer to Day 7 to see how you've improved!

Complete the following with your spouse in the order given, with proper form:

- [ ] 800-meter run as fast as you can (0.5 miles on treadmill)
- [ ] Rest 2 minutes.
- [ ] 2 minutes of as many air squats as possible
- [ ] Rest 1 minute.
- [ ] 2 minutes of as many push-ups as possible
- [ ] Rest 1 minute.
- [ ] 2 minutes of as many pendulum lunges as possible

DAY 18 WORKOUT

WARM-UP

- [ ] 400-meter jog (0.25 miles on treadmill)
- [ ] 10 walk-out/walk-ins
- [ ] 20 arm circles each direction
- [ ] 20 mountain-climbers (right/left is 1 rep)
- [ ] 15 air squats
- [ ] 16 bird dogs, holding each rep for 3 seconds (right/left is 1 rep)
- [ ] 10 burpees

WORKOUT

Complete the following workout as fast as you can with proper form. Both partners work simultaneously.

4 rounds:

- [ ] 16 bent-over dumbbell rows
- [ ] 18 dumbbell thrusters
- [ ] 20 partner Russian twists with kettlebell oblique twist (one rep is when both partners have twisted with the kettlebell.)
- [ ] Do 10 reps facing one direction and the last 10 facing the opposite direction.

DAY 19 WORKOUT

WARM-UP

- [ ] 400-meter jog (0.5 miles)
- [ ] 20 lateral lunges (10 each leg)
- [ ] 20 stationary lunges (10 each leg)
- [ ] 20 high kicks
- [ ] 10 slow air squats (lower for 5 seconds and hold at the bottom for 5 seconds)
- [ ] 10 air squats, regular pace
- [ ] 60-second plank
- [ ] 30-second side plank, right
- [ ] 30-second side plank, left

WORKOUT

Set a timer for 20 minutes and perform as many rounds as you can of the following circuit:

- [ ] 20 partner med ball squat passes (10 passes each partner)
- [ ] 20 partner med ball sit-ups
- [ ] 20 partner med ball standing oblique passes
- [ ] 400-meter run (0.25 miles on treadmill)

DAY 20—REST DAY

DAY 21 WORKOUT

WARM-UP

- [ ] 400-meter jog (0.25 miles on treadmill)
- [ ] 20 world's greatest stretch (10 each side)
- [ ] 30 mock kettlebell swings
- [ ] 20 air squats
- [ ] 20 butt kicks
- [ ] 20 squat pulses

WORKOUT

Set a timer and perform the following as fast as you can, using proper form, of course! Only one partner works at a time; the other partner rests until it's his or her turn. Each partner must complete the given number of repetitions.

5 rounds:

- [ ] 10 tuck jumps
- [ ] 12 goblet squats with kettlebell
- [ ] 14 Russian kettlebell swings

After you finish this, time yourselves as you run 800 meters (0.5 miles on treadmill) together, as fast as you can.

DAY 22 WORKOUT

WARM-UP

- ☐ 400-meter jog
- ☐ 10 walk-out/walk-ins
- ☐ 20 arm circles each direction
- ☐ 30 Russian twists
- ☐ 30 jumping jacks
- ☐ 20 wall push-ups

WORKOUT

Set a timer for 20 minutes and perform as many rounds as you can of the following circuit:

- ☐ 12 partner push-ups with shoulder tap
- ☐ 12 burpee jump-overs (6 jumps per partner)
- ☐ 12 dumbbell push-press (12 per partner; each partner works simultaneously)
- ☐ 12 knee tucks (12 per partner; each partner works simultaneously)

DAY 23 WORKOUT

WARM-UP

- [ ] 50 jumping jacks
- [ ] 200-meter jog (0.12 miles on treadmill)
- [ ] 20 butt kicks
- [ ] 20 high knees
- [ ] 20 high kicks
- [ ] 20 lateral lunges (10 each leg)
- [ ] 20 wall push-ups
- [ ] 20 arm circles each direction

BENCHMARK WORKOUT

*Record your scores for each section of this workout and compare them to your scores from days 7 and 17!

Complete the following with your spouse in the order given, with proper form:

- [ ] 800-meter run as fast as you can (0.5 miles on treadmill)
- [ ] Rest 2 minutes
- [ ] 2 minutes of as many air squats as possible
- [ ] Rest 1 minute
- [ ] 2 minutes of as many push-ups as possible
- [ ] Rest 1 minute
- [ ] 2 minutes of as many pendulum lunges as possible

DAY 24—REST DAY

Great job! You completed your month's work of tough partner workouts! I hope you and your spouse had fun and enjoyed pushing and motivating one another, especially on days when working out was the last thing either of you wanted to do! I hope that, in the end, you were glad you exercised and that you feel fitter, stronger, and closer to each other as a result.

If you're not ready for the sweat sessions to end, I encourage you to keep up the habit! Reach out to a nearby gym or invest in more gym equipment to ensure that you keep progressing. You can even revisit the workouts of this book, making them more difficult by using heavier weights, and/or by performing more reps and for longer periods of time.

Please feel free to reach out to me on social media for any workout tips! You can find me on Instagram at @dianaandersontyler and on Twitter *@dandersontyler*. Connect with our CrossFit gym, CrossFit 925, at *facebook.com/crossfit925* for motivation, workouts, and nutrition tips!

On behalf of Ben and myself, thank you so much for embarking on this journey of spiritual and physical fitness with us. We pray that you've been blessed and encouraged and trust that God will continue to build you two up as you love and serve one another as Christ loves and serves His bride, the Church.

Stay fit, stay faithful,

"And I am certain that God, who began the good work within you, will continue his work until it is finally finished on the day when Christ Jesus returns."

—*Philippians 1:6, NLT*

APPENDIX A
EXERCISE INSTRUCTIONS

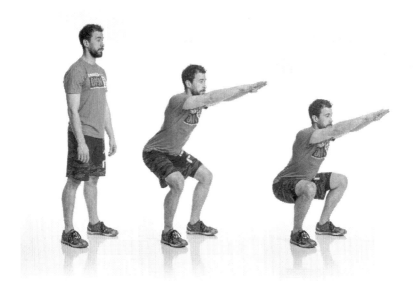

AIR SQUAT

1. Stand with your feet spread apart at a distance slightly wider than the shoulders. Position your feet so that your toes angle out. This angle varies from person to person, but should be about 30 degrees. Keep your weight on the heels to prevent yourself from rolling up onto the balls of your feet.

2. Keep your chest up, shoulders back, head up. This helps promote a nice, safe, intact lumbar curve.

3. Place arms straight out in front of your chest. The arms should be in a comfortable position as they act as counter balance to the motion of the exercise.

4. Bend your knees as you lower yourself down. Pretend there is a chair behind you that you're reaching back to sit on. Your knees should track over your feet and never jut out over them. In other words, your knees should be pointing in the same direction as your toes. If you find your knees starting to cave in, focus on pushing them out. A good way to achieve this is by imagining you are tearing the floor apart with your feet.

5. The push back up should be generated from your hamstrings and glutes. Your chest and head should remain pointing straight forward. As you rise, your arms will probably lower back to your sides naturally. Make sure your knees keep tracking with your toes and do not begin to buckle inwards. Also be sure to keep your lumbar curve intact (curved). Generally speaking, if you have your chest and head up, your lumbar curve will be in the correct position.

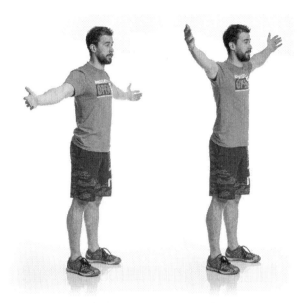

ARM CIRCLES
(FORWARD AND BACKWARD)

1. Stand in a neutral position with feet hip-width apart. Your arms should be straight out to the sides so your body forms a "T."

2. Begin making slow circles in a forward motion with your arms, then gradually make larger ones and complete the given number of repetitions.

3. Repeat in the opposite direction.

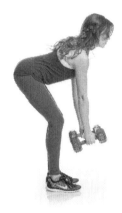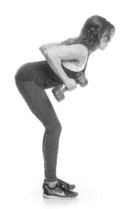

BENT-OVER DUMBBELL ROW

1. Stand with knees bent and your torso at a sixty degree angle.

2. With the weights fully extended straight down in your hands, bring them straight up to your chest, contracting your shoulder blades fully.

3. Slowly return to the starting position.

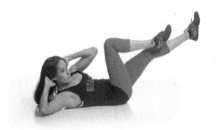 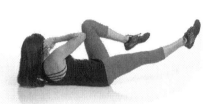

BICYCLE CRUNCH

1. Lie face up on the floor and lace your fingers behind your head. Keep elbows back.

2. Bring knees in toward your chest and lift shoulder blades off the ground without pulling on your neck.

3. Straighten the left leg out while simultaneously twisting upper body to the right, bringing the left elbow towards the right knee.

4. Switch sides, bringing right elbow towards the left knee.

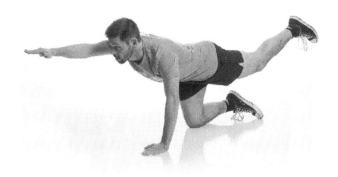

BIRD DOG

1. Kneel on the floor with hands firmly placed about shoulder width apart.

2. Brace your abs and point one arm out straight in front as you extend the opposite leg behind you. Squeeze your glutes and keep your abs tight.

3. Hold for three seconds and then switch sides.

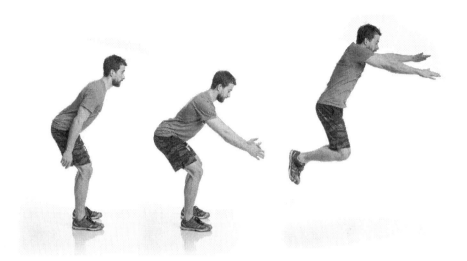

BROAD JUMP

1. Perform an air squat (see description of "Air Squat").

2. At the bottom position of the squat, swing your arms back and extend your knees and hips to jump powerfully forward.

3. Land softly and quietly on the mid-foot, rolling into the heels. You should be in a squat position. Repeat for the given number of reps.

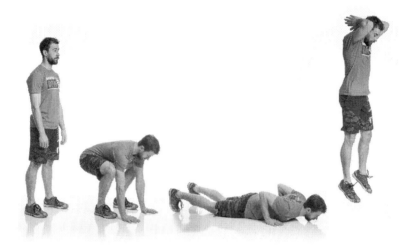

BURPEE

1. Lower your body down using proper squat form. Place hands on the ground in front of you.

2. Jump your feet back to a plank position, then quickly lower your chest to the ground.

3. Push yourself back up to a plank position and jump your feet back in toward your hands..

4. Jump back up and simultaneously clap your hands behind your head. Stand up all the way, extending the hips fully before beginning your next rep.

NOTE: To modify this exercise, you may eliminate the push-up component. To further modify for beginners, you may also walk your feet out and back in instead of jumping them out and in.

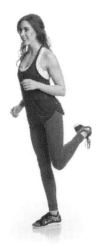 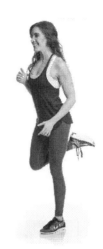

BUTT KICKS

1. Begin by jogging normally, either in place or traveling for a short distance.

2. Then begin raising your heels up toward your bottom as you jog, using rapid, forceful movements. Again, you may either do these in place or traveling.

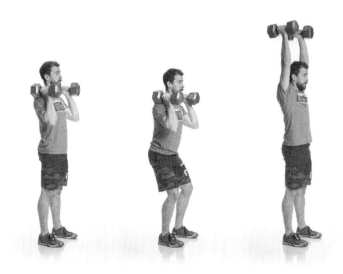

DUMBBELL PUSH-PRESS

1. Stand holding a pair of dumbbells just outside of your shoulders with arms bent and palms facing each other. Feet should be hip-width apart.

2. Dip your knees slightly then explosively push up through your legs, driving your arms upward at the same time. Make sure your biceps are by your ears in the overhead position.

3. Return the dumbbells to your shoulders and repeat.

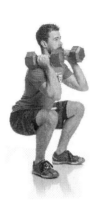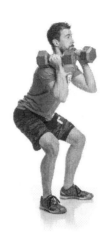

DUMBBELL THRUSTER

1. Hold a pair of dumbbells in front of your shoulders with bent elbows. Feet should be in your squat stance (see the description for "Air Squats" above).

2. Initiate the squat by pushing your hips back, then bend your knees as you lower yourself down as in a normal squat. Make sure your torso remains upright. Do not allow the dumbbells to pull you forward .

3. As your return to a standing position, explosively press the dumbbells overhead. Make sure your biceps are by your ears in the overhead position and that your legs are straight.

4. Lower the dumbbells to your shoulders and repeat for the given number of repetitions.

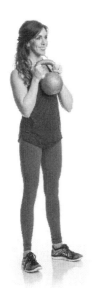
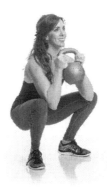

GOBLET SQUAT WITH KETTLEBELL

1. Hold a kettlebell by its horns at your chest. Stand with feet shoulder-width apart, torso upright.

2. With the kettlebell against your chest, squat down with the goal of having your elbows slide down along the inside of your knees. It's okay to have the elbows push the knees out a bit as you descend. Focus on keeping your back flat.

3. Rise out of the squat by driving through your heels.

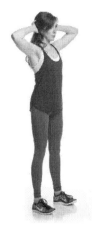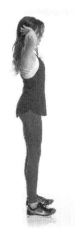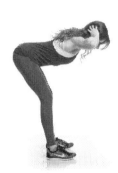

GOOD-MORNING

1. Begin with hands behind your head, fingers interlaced. Keep your shoulder blades pinched together and your knees slightly bent.

2. Begin by bending at your hips, moving them back as you bend over to near parallel. Keep your lower back arched.

3. Reverse the motion by extending through the hips with your glutes and hamstrings. Continue until you have returned to the starting position.

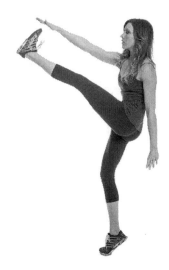

HIGH KICKS

1. Stand up straight with your kicking leg just behind your planted leg.

2. Kick your leg in front of you. Take it up as high as it will go while maintaining a straight spine as much as possible.

3. Return to the starting position, and repeat on the opposite side. You may do these in place or traveling.

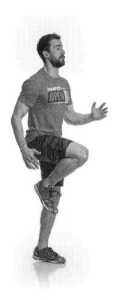

HIGH KNEES

1. Begin jogging, either in place or over a short distance.

2. Drive one knee up toward your chest and quickly return it to the ground. Follow immediately with the opposite knee.

3. Continue alternating for the given number of repetitions.

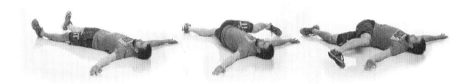

IRON CROSS

1. Lie on your back with your legs straight in front of you.

2. Bring one leg straight into the air, then bring it across your body so it rests on the ground.

3. Hold for 3-5 seconds, then repeat on the opposite side.

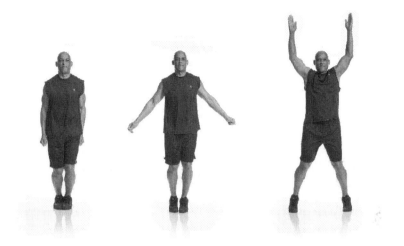

JUMPING JACK

1. Begin by standing feet together with arms at your sides.

2. Bend your knees and jump, moving your feet apart until they are wider than shoulder width. (You should be on the balls of your feet.) At the same time, raise your arms all the way overhead.

3. Maintain a slight bend in your knees as you jump your feet back together and return your arms to your sides. Repeat for the given number of reps.

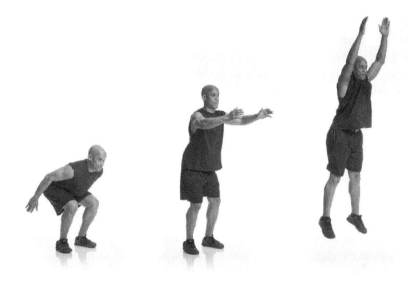

JUMP SQUAT

1. Refer to the "Air Squat" description.

2. Jump explosively to rise out of the squatting position.

3. With control, land in a squat position to complete one rep.

NOTE: Remember not to let your knees jut over your toes or let them cave inward as you jump.

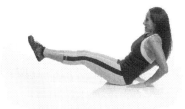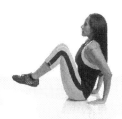

KNEE TUCK

1. Sit on the floor with hands just behind your hips. Legs are outstretched in front of you.

2. Keeping your torso fixed, lengthen and lift your legs so that your feet are at about chest level.

3. Keeping heels out, use your abs to draw your knees in toward your chest.

NOTE: To make this more challenging, bend your elbows, lowering your back toward the floor. To make this easier, decrease the range of motion so your knees remain bent throughout the movement.

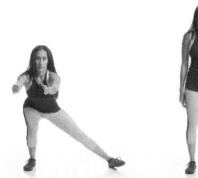
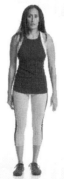
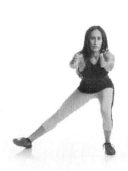

LATERAL LUNGE

1. Stand with your feet hip-width apart and make sure you have about two to three feet of space on either side of you.

2. Step sideways a comfortable distance, 2 or 3 feet, with one leg. Plant the heel of the lunging foot and keep the foot of the non-lunging leg pointed forward.

3. Sit back into the lunging leg to create a definite crease in your hip. Keep your weight in the heel.

4. Push off the heel of the lunging foot to bring feet together to the standing position. Repeat on opposite side and alternate for given number of repetitions.

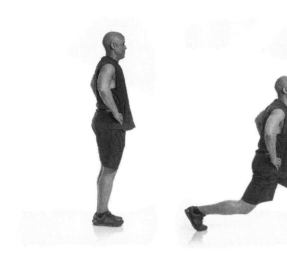

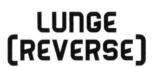

LUNGE
(REVERSE)

1. Stand with feet shoulder-width apart, torso upright with arms hanging straight at your sides.

2. Take a slow, controlled lunge backward with your right foot.

3. Lower your hips so that your front, left leg becomes parallel to the floor. At this point your left knee should be positioned directly over your ankle and your left foot should be pointing straight ahead. Your right knee should be bent at a 90-degree angle and pointing toward the floor. Your right heel should be lifted.

4. Push through both feet to straighten your legs. Bring your left foot back to meet your right in the starting position. Repeat on the other side, and continue alternating for the given number of repetitions.

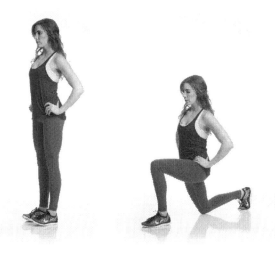

LUNGE
(WALKING AND STATIONARY)

1. Stand with feet shoulder-width apart, torso upright with arms hanging straight at your sides.

2. Take a slow, controlled lunge forward with one foot. As you lunge, lower your body and allow the lunging knee to bend until your thigh is parallel to the ground.

3. If performing a stationary lunge, push explosively off the lunging foot to return to the starting position. If performing walking lunges, push through the heel of the lunging foot to bring the back foot to meet it.

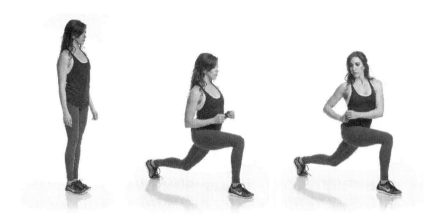

LUNGE WITH TWIST OVER LUNGING KNEE

1. Stand with feet shoulder-width apart, torso upright with arms hanging straight at your sides.

2. Take a slow, controlled lunge forward with one foot. As you lunge, lower your body and allow the lunging knee to bend until your thigh is parallel to the ground.

3. In the lunge position, bend your elbows at ninety degrees and rotate your torso in the direction of your bent knee.

4. If performing walking lunges, push through the heel of the lunging foot to bring the back foot to meet it.

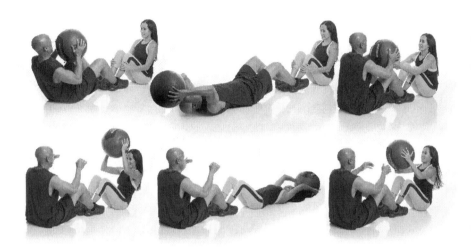

MED BALL SIT-UP

1. Position yourself opposite your partner and lie on the floor. Place your toes against your partner's toes.

2. Partner One holds the med ball at his or her chest and performs a sit-up, reaching the ball over his or head until it touches the floor. Partner Two performs a sit-up at the same time.

3. As Partner One sits up, he or she passes the ball to Partner Two who then performs a sit-up with the med ball. Repeat for the given number of repetitions.

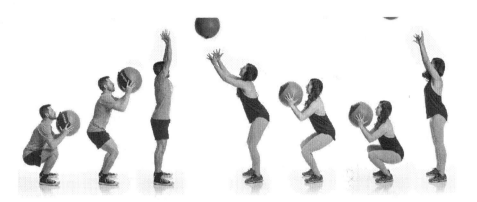

MED BALL SQUAT PASS

1. Stand facing your partner, about six to eight feet apart.

2. Partner One takes the med ball, holds it at his or her chest, and performs a squat.

3. As Partner One stands, he or she uses his legs and shoulders to drive the ball up, sending it high into the air.

4. Partner Two catches the ball as he or she squats, and repeats the movement.

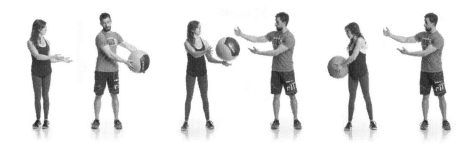

MED BALL STANDING OBLIQUE PASS

1. Stand six to eight feet away from your partner. Each of you face the same direction.

2. Partner One takes the med ball and twists to the outside.

3. As Partner One twists back around, he or she throws the ball to Partner Two.

4. Partner Two catches the ball, then twists to the outside and passes it back to Partner One, repeating the movement.

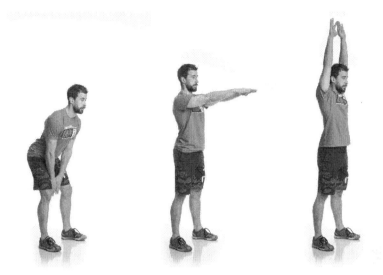

MOCK KETTLEBELL SWINGS

1. Assume an air squat stance with feet shoulder-width apart, toes angled out slightly.

2. Keeping your chest lifted and your lower back arched, reach down to the floor with your fingertips.

3. Thrust your hips forward as you stand from the squat position. Your arms should be straight, as if your hands are holding an invisible weight.

4. Swing your arms overhead until your biceps are beside your ears.

5. Squat to lower your arms back down toward the floor.

NOTE: Fully extend your hips (a.k.a., "open up" your hips) when you stand.

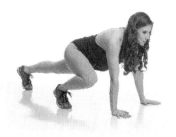 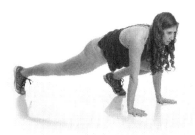

MOUNTAIN-CLIMBER

1. Place your hands on the floor, slightly wider than shoulder width. Step out with your feet to assume a plank position with arms extended.

2. While holding your upper body in place, alternate bringing the right and left knees toward your chest.

3. Keep your hips down and increase the intensity by performing the movement faster as you feel comfortable.

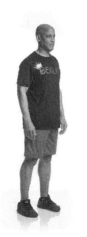
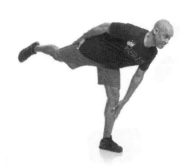

OПE-LEGGED
ROMAПIAП DEADLIFT

1. Stand with feet shoulder-width apart and lift one foot a few inches off the floor.

2. Keep your back straight and the torso tight. Look straight ahead. Pull your shoulder blades back.

3. Lower the upper body by bending at the hips. Keep the back straight.

4. Pretending you have a weight in your hand, slide your hand in front of the thigh and shin of your supporting leg. Push the hips back and slightly bend your knee during the descent.

5. Swing the free leg back so it stays in line with the torso.

6. Lower the upper body until a mild stretch is felt in the hamstrings.

7. Return to the starting position and repeat for the given number of reps.

168 PERFECT FIT· COUPLES EDITION

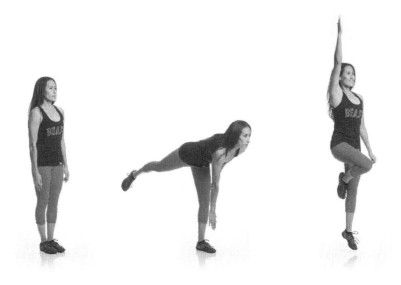

ONE-LEGGED ROMANIAN DEADLIFT WITH ONE-LEGGED HOP

1. Follow the instructions given for the One-Legged Romanian deadlift, but each time you return to the starting position, pull your abs in and hop a few inches off the floor with your non-working leg.

2. As you jump, extend the same arm as jumping leg to the ceiling.

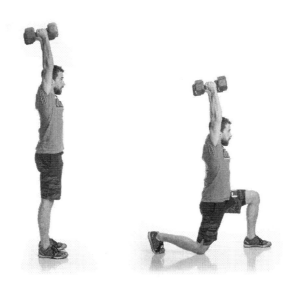

OVERHEAD WALKING LUNGE WITH DUMBBELLS

1. Hold a pair of dumbbells overhead, arms fully extended with biceps by your ears. Stand with feet shoulder-width apart.

2. Take a slow, controlled lunge forward with one foot. As you lunge, lower your body and allow the lunging knee to bend until your thigh is parallel to the ground. Keep arms strong and locked out overhead. Do not let elbows bend.

3. If performing walking lunges, push through the heel of the lunging foot to bring the back foot to meet it.

PARTNER BURPEE

1. Partner One stands with arms raised overhead.

2. Partner Two performs a burpee and "high fives" both of Partner One's hands as both partners do the jump portion of the burpee.

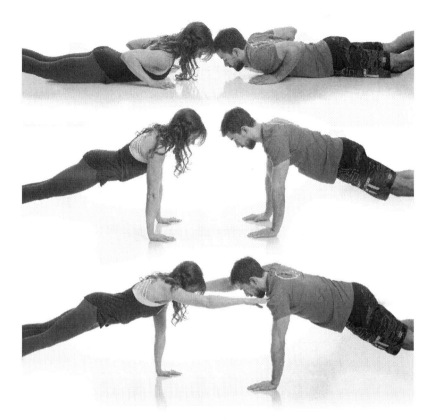

PARTNER PUSH-UP
WITH SHOULDER TAP

1. Face your spouse in your preferred push-up position (see below for instructions on modified and traditional push-ups).

2. Perform a push-up at the same time as your spouse.

3. When you push up, reach across with your right hand and tap your spouse's left shoulder.

4. Push up again, then reach across with your left hand to tap your spouse's right shoulder.

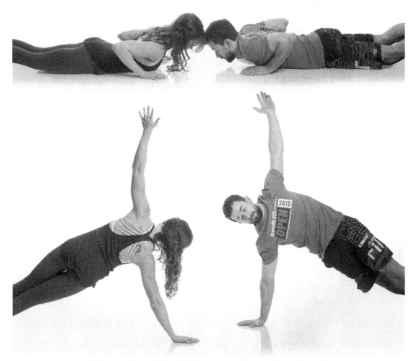

PARTNER PUSH-UP
WITH REACH

1. Face your spouse in your preferred push-up position (see below for instructions on modified and traditional push-ups).

2. Perform a push-up at the same time as your spouse.

3. At the top of the push-up, rotate your torso to the right while bringing your right hand off the floor. Lift your right arm up to the ceiling, feeling a stretch through your chest as you gaze toward your fingertips. Hold for 3 seconds, then return your hand to the floor to complete another repetition.

4. Repeat on the opposite side.

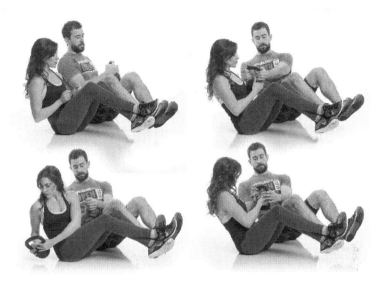

PARTNER RUSSIAN TWISTS

1. Follow the instructions given for "Russian Twist" below.

2. When doing this with your spouse, sit side by side and simply pass the kettlebell to one another. Do half the reps facing one direction and the next half facing the opposite direction.

PENDULUM LUNGE

1. Perform a forward lunge, immediately followed by a reverse lunge on the same leg. See the instructions for these above.

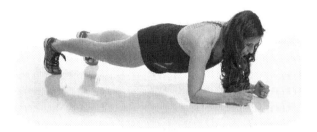

PLANK

1. Get into a standard push-up position, and then lower yourself onto your forearms. Elbows should be aligned below your shoulders, and arms parallel to your body at about shoulder-width distance.

2. Keep your core tight, bellybutton pulled in toward your spine as you hold this position.

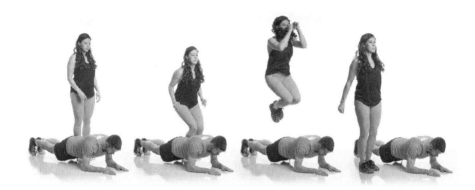

PLANK-AND-JUMP

1. Partner One holds a forearm plank.

2. Partner Two stands parallel to Partner One and jumps laterally over Partner One's body.

3. Partner Two jumps back and forth for the given number of repetitions before switching with Partner One.

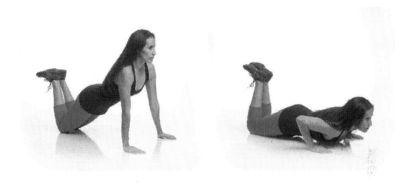

PUSH-UP (MODIFIED)

1. Get into a hands-and-knees position on a mat or floor. Hands should be slightly wider than shoulder-width apart, fingers facing forward.

2. Keeping your core (abdominals and back) tight, slowly lower yourself in a straight line. Make sure your neck stays neutral, naturally aligned with your spine. Don't let your hips pike up in the air or your lower back sag.

3. Continue to lower yourself until your chest touches the mat or floor or, for beginners, your arms form a 90-degree angle.

4. Keeping your spine rigid and tummy pulled in, press your hands into the floor to return to start position.

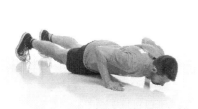 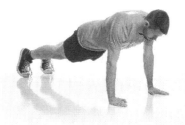

PUSH-UPS (TRADITIONAL)

1. Get into a plank position on the ground: hands and feet slightly wider than shoulder-width apart.

2. Keeping your core (abdominals and back) tight, slowly lower yourself in a straight line. Make sure your neck stays neutral, naturally aligned with your spine. Don't let your hips pike up in the air or your lower back sag.

3. Continue to lower yourself until your chest touches the mat or floor or, for beginners, your arms form a ninety-degree angle.

4. Keeping your spine rigid and abdominals pulled in, press your hands into the floor to return to start position.

NOTE: Think about exploding powerfully from the bottom position to increase the intensity of this movement.

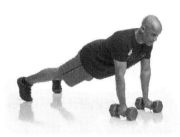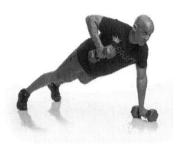

RENEGADE ROW

1. Place a pair of dumbbells side by side on the floor. Then get into a plank position with hands gripping either dumbbell, feet hip-width apart. Make sure dumbbells are about shoulder-width apart.

2. Bend your right elbow and pull the dumbbell until your elbow passes your torso. Keep the elbow tight and close to your body. Keep abdominals engaged and neck in a neutral position. Press the left dumbbell into the floor for balance.

3. Lower your arm and repeat on the opposite side.

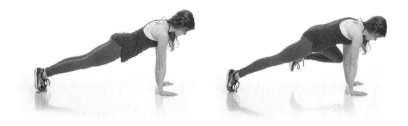

REPTILE

1. Assume a push-up position.

2. Keeping core tight, bring your right knee toward your right tricep.

3. Return foot to the floor and repeat on the opposite side.

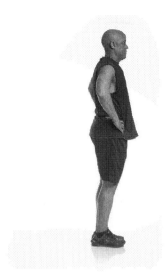
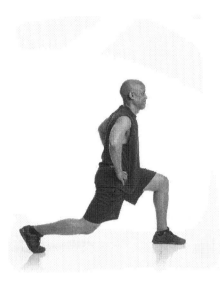

REVERSE LUNGE

1. Stand with feet shoulder-width apart, torso upright with arms hanging straight at your sides.

2. Take a slow, controlled lunge backward with one foot. As you lunge, lower your body and allow the lunging knee to bend until your thigh is parallel to the ground.

3. Keeping your abs pulled in and pressing your forward heel into the floor, step forward to a standing position.

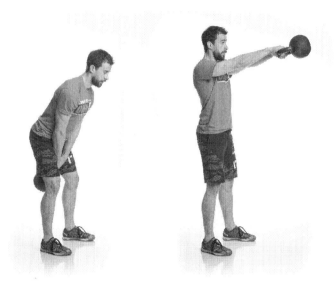

RUSSIAN KETTLEBELL SWING

1. Hold a kettlebell (start with a light one until you're comfortable with the movement) with both hands in front of you. Stand in a squat position with feet shoulder-width apart, toes angled out slightly.

2. Lean over slightly at your waist and bend your knees as if to do a partial squat. Keep your lower back tight and arched, and keep head facing forward. Do not look down.

3. Swing the kettlebell up to eye level with an explosive hip thrust.

4. Reverse the motion to return the kettlebell to the starting position between your legs, and immediately begin the next swing.

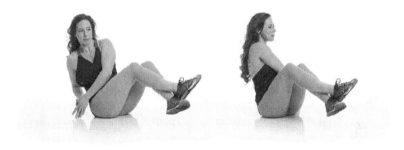

RUSSIAN TWIST

1. Sit on the floor. Lift your feet off the floor a few inches and cross your ankles.

2. Keeping your core tight, twist to one side, bringing your hands toward your hip. Repeat on the opposite side.

Russian Twist with Kettlebell

1. Sit on the floor holding a kettlebell at your chest. Lift your feet off the floor a few inches and cross your ankles.

2. Keeping your core tight, twist to one side, bringing the kettlebell toward your hip. Repeat on the opposite side.

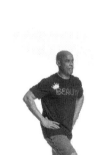 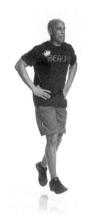 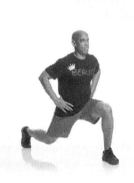

SCISSOR JUMP

1. Assume a lunge-stance position with one foot forward with your knee bent. The rear knee should almost be touching the ground.

2. Make sure that the front knee is over the midline of the foot.

3. Extending through both legs, jump as high as you can, swinging your arms to help you.

4. As you jump, switch the position of your legs in midair, moving your front leg to the back and the rear leg to the front.

5. As you land, absorb the impact through the legs by assuming the lunge position. Then repeat.

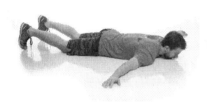 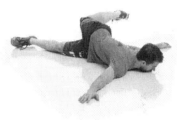

SCORPION

1. Lie face-down on a mat or on the floor. Stretch your arms out to either side, forming a T.

2. Lift your left leg away from the floor as far as you can, then move it to the right, crossing it over your right leg. As you do this, twist your hips to the right, allowing the left leg to touch the ground on the right side.

3. Return your left leg back to starting position and repeat the movement with your right leg.

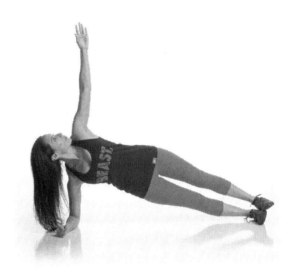

SIDE PLANK

1. Lie on your left side with your knees straight.

2. Prop your upper body up on your left elbow and forearm.

3. Lift your hips until your body forms a straight line from your ankles to your shoulders. Feet are stacked on top of each another.

4. Pull your bellybutton in and keep your chest high and hip lifting toward the ceiling.

5. Extend top arm straight up into the air.

NOTE: To make this movement easier, you can place the top foot a few inches in front of the bottom one, or drop to your knees and place them on top of each other. Make sure your hips don't sag!

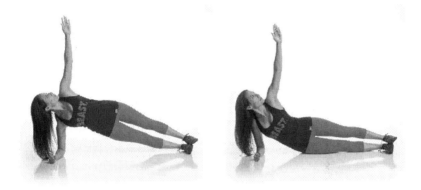

SIDE PLANK HIP DIP

1. Follow the instructions for the side plank above.
2. Slowly lower your hip until it barely grazes the floor.
3. Shoot the hip back up to the start position.

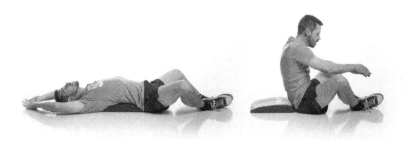

SIT-UPS

1. Grab your rolled-up towel or AbMat and place it above your waistband, against your tailbone.

2. Lie on your back with arms overhead and feet in a butterfly position (soles of feet touching).

3. Take a breath in and forcefully "throw" your arms over your body as you sit up.

4. Touch your shoes as you exhale and return to a lying position, keeping the arms straight. Make sure your shoulder blades touch the floor at the bottom to achieve the full range of motion.

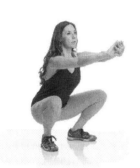 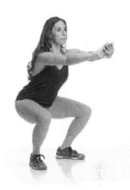

SQUAT PULSE

1. Perform an air squat, but instead of standing all the way up, use your glutes to lift only a few inches.

2. Repeat this pulsing motion for the given number of reps.

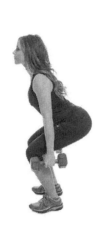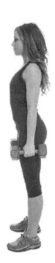

SUITCASE DEADLIFT

1. Hold one dumbbell to the side of your body. Feet are hip-width apart.

2. With shoulders back, chest lifted, and lower back in a natural arch, being lowering your body by pushing your hips back. Then bend your knees and continue moving your rear back while maintaining the arch in your lower back.

3. The dumbbell should be lowering in a straight path in line with your shoulder blades. When you lose the natural curve in your spine and begin to round your back, stop lowering and reverse the motion.

4. To initiate the lift, use your glute muscles to powerfully thrust your hips forward. Focus on keeping your torso level and not leaning or twisting toward the dumbbell.

NOTE: As your flexibility and mobility increases, you can lower the dumbbell more and more until you can touch the floor.

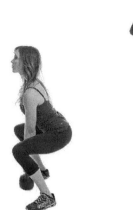
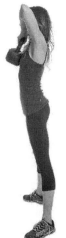
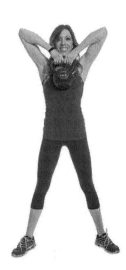

SUMO DEADLIFT HIGH PULL

1. Stand with feet slightly wider than your squat stance. The kettlebell should be in line with the balls of your feet on the ground.

2. Drop your hips and keep arms straight to grab onto the kettlebell.

3. Keeping your lower back arched and tight and chest up, use power from your legs and hips to drive the kettlebell to a top position right under your chin. Your elbows should be high, as if to form a "V" shape around your face.

4. Release your arms, bend your knees, and keep your chest high and facing forward to return to the starting position.

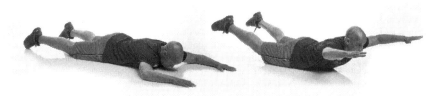

SUPERMAN

1. Lie face down on a soft surface with arms extended overhead. Keep your neck in a neutral position.

2. Keeping your arms and legs straight (not locked) and torso stationary, lift your arms and legs towards the ceiling as if to form a "U" with your body.

3. Hold arms and legs a few inches off the floor for 1 to 2 seconds and gently lower.

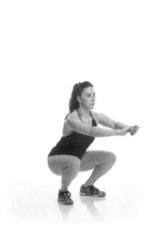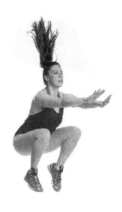

TUCK JUMP

1. Perform a jump squat, but as you jump, bring your knees up, "tucking" them as close to your chest as possible.

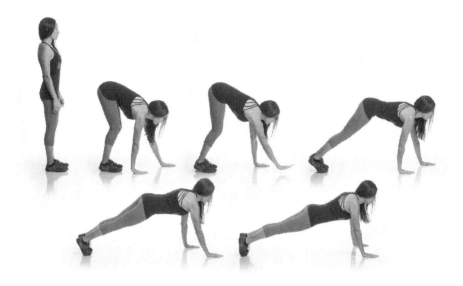

WALK-OUT/WALK-IN

1. Begin in a standing position. Bend over to touch your toes and walk your hands out until you are in a plank position.

2. Walk the hands back in to your feet keeping legs as straight as possible, and repeat for the given number of repetitions.

WALL PUSH-UP

1. Face a wall, standing an arm's length away. Feet are slightly apart, legs straight with weight in your toes.

2. Place your hands on the wall so that hands are just outside shoulder width and are even with your chest.

3. Bend elbows about 90 degrees and lower body toward the wall without touching it.

4. Straighten arms and return to the starting position.

NOTE: To make this more difficult, move your feet farther away from the wall.

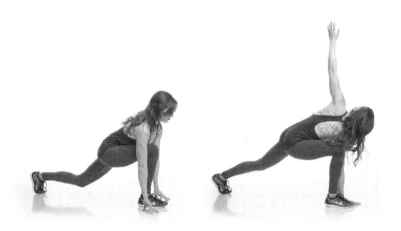

WORLD'S GREATEST STRETCH

1. Begin in a deep lunge. This will look like a 40-yard dash stance with hands on either side of your feet.

2. Keep your front hip, knee, and ankle aligned.

3. Rotate your torso to the right and lift your right arm up as high as you can, feeling a stretch through your chest and upper back.

4. Focus on maintaining balance by keeping your bellybutton pulled in and breathing steadily.

5. Keep back leg as straight as possible by firing your quads and glutes.

6. Hold for five seconds and then rotate to the left.

APPENDIX B
THE STRETCHES

Be sure to take time (5 to 10 minutes) to stretch at the end of every workout, focusing on the muscles most emphasized that day, as well as any areas that feel particularly tight or sore.

Stretching improves circulation, increases flexibility, helps maximize the range of motion in your joints, and reduces soreness and stress! Each stretch should be held between fifteen and thirty seconds and should feel good. If it becomes painful, ease up a bit, breathe deep, and go slower.

BACK EXTENSION

1. Lie on your stomach.
2. Prop yourself up on your elbows, extending your back.
3. Begin straightening your elbows, pressing your hands against the floor, until a gentle stretch is felt.

CALVES STRETCH

1. Place both hands on wall with arms extended.
2. Lean against wall with one leg bent forward and other leg extended back with knee straight and foot positioned directly forward.
3. Press rear heel into the floor and move hips slightly forward.
4. Hold and repeat on other leg.

CHEST AND SHOULDERS

1. Standing, interlock fingers behind your back, arms straight.
2. Keeping hands together, lift them as high as you comfortably can.
3. Hold for at least fifteen seconds.

HIP/GLUTE

1. Cross your left foot over right knee.
2. Grasp hands behind right thigh and gently pull thigh towards you, keeping the body relaxed.
3. Hold for at least fifteen seconds before switching sides.

INNER THIGH

1. Sit on the floor with feet pressed together.
2. Keep abs pulled in as you lean forward.
3. Keep leaning until you feel a nice stretch in your inner thighs.

LYING HAMSTRING STRETCH

1. Lie on the floor with your knees bent.

2. Straighten one leg up towards the ceiling and slowly pull it towards you, clasping your hands behind the thigh, calf, or ankle—whichever is most comfy.

3. Keep knee slightly bent. Hold for at least fifteen seconds before switching sides.

LYING QUAD STRETCH

1. Lie on your side and grasp your ankle.

2. Gently pull your ankle toward your butt, keeping your hips stable.

ONE-ARM CHEST STRETCH

1. Stand against the wall. While facing the wall, raise your right hand out to your side at chest height, palm against the wall.

2. Turn your body toward the left, away from the wall and your extended arm, until you feel a stretch.

3. Hold, switch sides, and repeat.

SEATED HAMSTRING STRETCH

1. Sit on the floor and extend one leg out straight.

2. Bend the other leg at the knee and position the sole of that foot against your opposite inner thigh.

3. Extend your arms and reach forward over the straight leg by bending at the waist as far as possible.

4. Hold, switch legs, and repeat.

SPINE TWIST

1. Lie on the floor and place your right foot on left knee.

2. Using your left hand, gently pull your right knee towards the floor, twisting your spine, keeping hips and shoulders on the floor, left arm straight out.

3. Hold for at least fifteen seconds before switching sides.

STANDING QUAD STRETCH

1. Grab a stationary object, like a chair, for balance with one hand.
2. Use the opposite hand to grasp the leg around the ankle, lifting it towards the buttocks.
3. Keep your back straight.
4. Hold, switch legs, and repeat.

TRICEPS

1. Standing, bend your right elbow behind your head and use your left hand to gently pull the right elbow in farther until you feel a stretch in the back of your arm (tricep).
2. Hold for at least fifteen seconds before switching sides.

UPPER BACK

1. Clasp your hands together in front of your chest, arms straight.
2. Round your back towards the floor, pressing your arms away from your body to feel a stretch in your upper back.
3. Hold for at least fifteen seconds.

ACKNOWLEDGEMENTS

Above all, Ben and I give all glory and praise to our Heavenly Father. It is only because of His strength and faithfulness that our marriage has been made stronger day by day and that this book has been written. We thank Him for sending His Son, Jesus Christ, to take our place on the cross and replace our sin-stained rags with His radiant righteousness. Without Him, we can do nothing (John 15:5).

Thank you so much to mighty superheroes George and Rachel Range and swing dance superstars Heidi Luong and Daniel Fryar for gracing this book with your mad modeling skills! I couldn't ask for better friends to pretend work out with!

Thank you, once again, to John McBrayer for being the best and most fun photographer in the world! You make fitness look glam! Check out his breathtaking portfolio at *johnmcbrayer.com.*

Thank you to Jeff and Joy Miller of Five Js Design for making this book beautiful inside and out, and for your infinite patience with this scatterbrained writer over the years!

A humongous "thank you!!!" to my gracious and big-hearted father-in-law, David, for patiently and expertly editing the rough draft and encouraging this writer's heart in no small way!

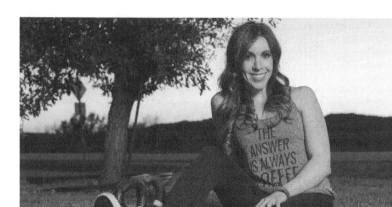

AUTHOR'S NOTE

Thank you so much for going on this journey of faith and fitness with Ben and me! I hope you enjoyed reading, praying, discussing, and sweating as much as we have! If you loved the book and have a moment to spare, we would really appreciate a short review online! Your help in spreading the word is greatly received.

Connect with us online!:
www.dianaandersontyler.com and *www.crossfit925.com*
Facebook.com/dianafit4faith and *Facebook.com/crossfit925*
Twitter *@dandersontyler*
Instagram *@dianaandersontyler* and *@crossfit925*

ABOUT THE AUTHORS

Diana Anderson-Tyler earned her degree in Radio-Television-Film from the University of Texas and her personal training certification from the Cooper Clinic in Dallas, Texas. She is also a Level 1 certified CrossFit coach. She's the author of five faith and fitness books for women, including *Fit for Faith: A Christian Woman's Guide to Total Fitness* and a memoir, *Immeasurable: Diving into the Depths of God's Love.* She is also a fiction writer and published her first inspirational fantasy novel, *Moonbow: The Colors of Iris,* last year.

Diana has been interviewed on *The 700 Club, The Harvest Show,* and has also been a guest on a number of radio broadcasts and podcasts. She currently writes entertainment and media-related articles for movieguide.org and contributes regularly to the health section of *charismamag.com.* Diana lives in San Antonio with her husband Ben where they own and coach at CrossFit 925, watch

Pixar and Marvel movies, and play Scrabble regularly. You can learn more at her website, *dianaandersontyler.com.*

Ben Tyler is a CrossFit Level 2 Coach and graduated from LeTourneau University in 2009 with a Bachelor of Science degree in Mechanical Engineering Technology. He became certified as a Level 1 CrossFit trainer in 2010 and coached at "Premier CrossFit" (*www.premiercrossfit.com*) in Tyler, Texas before moving to San Antonio. He completed the CrossFit Level 2 Certification in 2013.

An avid competitive swimmer, baseball player, and track athlete since age 7, power-lifter since age 14 and even a year or two in wrestling and football, Ben has been in athletics his entire life. He grew up doing any sport or fitness-related activity he could get his hands—or feet—on. Ben spent over a decade in the gym following different bodybuilding/conditioning routines until he found CrossFit. He hasn't looked back.

Ben loves steak, pizza, and coffee (added by me, Diana, without his permission, ha!).

Made in the USA
Columbia, SC
13 December 2019

84811282R00113